Heal Your Hips

Also by Lynda Huey

The Complete Waterpower Workout Book (with Robert Forster, P.T.)
The Waterpower Workout (with R. R. Knudson)
A Running Start: An Athlete, a Woman

Heal Your Hips

How to Prevent Hip Surgery— and What to Do If You Need It

Robert Klapper, M.D.
and
Lynda Huey

John Wiley & Sons, Inc.
New York • Chichester • Weinheim • Brisbane • Singapore • Toronto

Copyright © 1999 by Robert Klapper, M.D., and Lynda Huey. All rights reserved.
Published by John Wiley & Sons, Inc.
Published simultaneously in Canada.

The information contained in this book is not intended to serve as a replacement for professional medical advice. Any use of the information in this book is at the reader's discretion. The author and the publisher specifically disclaim any and all liability arising directly or indirectly from the use or application of any information contained in this book. A health care professional should be consulted regarding your specific situation.

The information contained in this book is not intended to be prescriptive. Any attempt to diagnose, treat, or rehabilitate an injury or disorder should come under the direction of a doctor, an orthopedic specialist, or a physical therapist. Before starting the exercises in this book, check with your doctor. Not all exercises are suitable for everyone. Anyone using these programs assumes the risk of injury from performing the exercises and/or using the equipment shown.

Library of Congress Cataloging-in-Publication Data:
Klapper, Robert.
    Heal your hips : how to prevent hip injury—and what to do if
you need it / Robert Klapper & Lynda Huey.
      p.   cm.
    ISBN 0-471-24997-1
    1. Hip joint—Popular works. 2. Hip joint—Surgery—Popular
works. I. Huey, Lynda. II. Title.
RD772.K53   1999
617.5'81—dc21   98-55120

Printed in the United States of America.
10 9 8 7

Contents

Preface

It was basketball great Wilt Chamberlain who, following his hip surgery, introduced Lynda Huey to me as "the most knowledgeable water trainer in the world." Lynda's and my collaboration has been terrific, because we are both passionate about our daily work, both committed to steering our patients to conservative care.

Here's how perfect a match we've been: Let's say you place a vibrating steel tuning fork, the density of which is 100 hertz, next to an 80-hertz tuning fork. The 80-hertz fork will remain silent. But if you bring close another tuning fork of 100 hertz, it will, without being struck, begin to vibrate. It has responded to the perfect match.

Lynda and I have been like those two tuning forks throughout the process of writing this book. We've taken turns inspiring and uplifting each other—keeping each other vibrating at 100 hertz. Lynda's notes for our book sparkled with the buoyant flow of body and water in her pool—her elixir of life. My own notes ran to dozens of pages about patients.

Many come to me because their doctors have flatly told them, "I'm the doctor, you're the patient." My answer: for me there's nothing better than patients who participate in getting themselves well. I'm delighted when they bring along popular articles on health and fitness to discuss during office visits or when they choose books to take home from my library. More power to them! And when we talk about their hips, I try to avoid jargon. I want to demystify their loss of mobility, their decreased strength, and loss of function. I use examples, anecdotes, X rays, quick drawings, and photographs as I encourage their understanding of the anatomy and physiology of a hip, that elegant piece of biological machinery.

"I *love* to operate," I say after listening to patients describe their pain. "But I'd rather we exhaust all conservative care to get you back to health."

Back to golf, tennis, running, skiing, pickup basketball, beach volleyball, bicycling—so many of my patients have their return to sports as a goal. And back to construction work, driving a bus, managing a restaurant, repairing computers—these recent patients of mine have sought to regain strength and mobility for their jobs. Most of my diagnoses lead to treatment in a pool, where those with arthritis, congenital hip problems, rheumatoid arthritis, and even more complicated hip problems become instant athletes and unhobbled workers as they walk, run, push, pull, bend, squat, lunge, jump, and lift themselves easily. Indeed, they can practice all their moves in the glove of water that protects them from pain.

People call my office from around the country, and some even fly in for consultations or surgery. Patients who want to learn Lynda's pool program often do the same. But not everyone can come to California to visit us, so Lynda and I have written this book as the next best thing. *Heal Your Hips* gives you a chance to learn about your hips, seek a correct diagnosis, begin positive treatment, and do everything possible to prevent hip surgery.

Nothing could make us happier.

—Robert C. Klapper, M.D.
Beverly Hills, California

Twenty-five years ago I sprinted for one of America's fastest relay teams. Twenty years ago I coached college athletes. Fifteen years ago my athletic injuries and those of my Olympic athletes led us into a pool for water training. There we pioneered the use of exercising in water to sustain fitness. Water embraced and surrounded us as we went through the fitness programs that I soon compiled for my first book, *The Waterpower Workout.* What all of us thought at the time was that we'd simply found a way to stay in shape while injuries healed.

We didn't expect this added bounty: through our efforts in the pool, we were speeding the healing of injuries.

By the late 1980s, heros from many sports made headlines by using *Waterpower* for their amazing recoveries. Physical therapists across America began to add water exercising to their programs, and when the media turned a spotlight on my articles in national magazines and on my exercise video, I began a second book, this one to include water therapies: *The Complete Waterpower Workout Book*. The book led to my work with Mike Shapow, P.T. For him I toned down my programs, making them manageable for general patients, people far less physically capable than athletes. I devised easy exercises so those with serious disabilities could begin at their own level. Yet I always took my drive for excellence into the pool with me and my patients. I expected every one of them to strive for top fitness, flexibility, and good form—for optimum performance. I also expected many of them to add land exercises to their rehabilitation programs. These were devised and assigned to patients by Mike Shapow, my partner at Total Aquatic Rehab.

Dr. Robert Klapper and I met in 1993, shortly after he performed hip arthroscopy on my friend Wilt Chamberlain. I had helped Wilt with rehabilitation in his pool after each of his surgeries: hip, knee, and elbow. Wilt told Dr. Klapper of his intention to work with me in the water, and before long, Dr. Klapper was sending dozens of patients into my pool to *prevent* hip surgery. In turn I observed him at work in his operating room; together we studied X rays in a view box. I learned why my programs were successful: if patients regained strength and flexibility in the muscles surrounding the hip it wouldn't matter if the interior of the joint was normal. As long as patients could function in their daily lives without undue pain they wouldn't need surgery.

To share that concept with as many hip patients as possible, we undertook this book. No one wants to live disabled and in pain, and hip pain is especially troublesome, because it leads to inactivity, which leads to numerous other health problems that cause further misery. Our exercise programs have been astonishingly successful, sparing many of our patients the surgical procedures described in Chapters 11 and 12. We hope you will commit to the self-help to follow.

—*Lynda Huey*
Santa Monica, California

Acknowledgments

The following people contributed to the success of this book:

Mike Shapow, P.T., collaborated on Chapters 8 and 9.

David Rubenstein, M.D., collaborated on Chapter 4 and raided his teaching files to supply us with examples of X rays, CT scans, and MRIs.

Bridget Failner, R.N., the head nurse at Cedars-Sinai Hospital, provided much of the information in Chapter 13.

Pete Romano managed to squeeze in time to shoot our pool photos in the midst of also shooting the underwater sequences of *Armageddon* and *Lethal Weapon 4*.

Andrew Maksym courageously went into the operating room, the hospital, the examining room, and physical therapy clinics to handle our "guerilla" photography.

Joel Lipton shot the beautiful cover photos.

Marjory Kay drew the medical illustrations for us with insight and good humor.

Zan Knudson read the manuscript and helped make it a concise whole.

LaReine Chabut-Deerborn, Kevin O'Leary, D.C., Jean Shapiro, David Bell, Barbara Linton, Pattie O'Leary, PTA, Vince Newman, P.T., Lisa Nevis, P.T., Cec Schulman, Shelly Pepper, Karol Silverstein, Jim Birch, René Ruegg, John Buch, Livia Shemansky, Lucy Mazmanian, Vince Warren, Bill Belding, Paul Batchelor, and Tracey Maron-Anthony appeared for photo shoots.

Jennifer McGaw did photo editing.

Cedars-Sinai Hospital gave us permission to shoot photos in the operating room and a hospital room, and the staff received us graciously.

Earl Katz thought up the book's title.

Cybill Shepherd generously let us shoot cover photos in her backyard.

John Jericiau, P.T., read the physical therapy chapters and helped us shoot accurately the land exercise and hip precaution photos.

Lolly Krissman graciously offered us the use of her pool for the pool program photo shoot.

The staff of IntenseCity Sports Medicine and Rehabilitation and the staff of Dr. Klapper's office were most helpful in accommodating our photo shoots.

Leanne Marlier at Back to Work Physical Therapy let us shoot the SwimEx photo at her clinic.

Bibi Vabry, Mark Frantz, Zoila Fernandez, and Kitty Nolan in Dr. Klapper's office lent their assistance whenever needed.

Hilde Brooks, Pattie O'Leary, and Amy Okohira of Total Aquatic Rehab kept everything running smoothly while Director Lynda Huey went into book-writing seclusion.

Howard Bein exhibited fathomless patience while running the office of Huey's Athletic Network in a maelstrom.

Jane Jordan Browne was the glue in this project at key moments.

Speedo Authentic Fitness supplied the bathing suits.

Excel Sports Science supplied the unitards.

WaterWear supplied the bodysuit on the cover.

Vince Newman, P.T., and massage therapist Joe Daniel helped bring Lynda Huey's shoulder back from injury so she could go surfing with Dr. Klapper again.

Massage therapist (and extreme outdoorsman) Gary Ochman provided the bicycling terminology and offered advice on the massage therapy section.

The following orthopedic surgeons at the Hospital for Special Surgery in New York instructed Dr. Klapper in the field of hip surgery: Eduardo Salvati, M.D., Chit Ranawat, M.D., Philip Wilson, M.D., Paul Pellici, M.D., and Larry Dorr, M.D.

Orthopedic surgeon Robert Kerlan, M.D., of the Kerlan-Jobe Orthopedic Clinic, inspired Dr. Klapper to do his part in demystifying medicine for the lay public.

Leroy Perry Jr., D.C., a pioneer in the field of sports medicine and aquatic therapy, has been an inspiration to both Lynda Huey and Robert Klapper, M.D.

Kendall Corporation supplied the inflatable stockings used after implant surgery.

Dyonics, Inc. and Biomet, Inc. supplied the surgical instruments used in hip arthroscopy.

De Puy, Inc. supplied the implants used in hip implant surgery.

1

Ten Minutes in Water, Ten Minutes on Land

Your hip hurts, and you aren't quite sure what to do about it.

You've just come home from a long walk or bike ride and suddenly discover a deep ache. Or maybe for weeks your hip has been bothering you off and on. The pain keeps you awake at night. You're even starting to limp. Perhaps you were told years ago that you have a "hip condition" that was bound to be troublesome later in life. Now you fear your pain will go on forever.

Whether your hip pain is a surprise or a problem you've been expecting, you want relief. Here's how to get it. Go to your nearest swimming pool and do the ten-minute program that follows. The pain relief will be worth the effort of traveling to the water.

Ten-Minute Pool Program

Make a photocopy of the shaded box on the next page and laminate it to take to the pool with you. Place it poolside and follow the order of the exercises. Do each exercise for one minute.

While doing the exercises, focus on the physical abilities of your healthy and unhealthy hips. Notice whether you take a longer stride with one leg than with the other or whether you can lift one leg higher to the side.

Ten-Minute Pool Program

Exercise 1. Walking forward, backward, sideways

Exercise 2. Bouncing

Exercise 3. Bicycle Kick

Exercise 4. Hip Openers

Exercise 5. Leg Swings

Exercise 6. Internal and External Rotations

Exercise 7. Squats

Exercise 8. Lateral Split

Exercise 1. Shallow Water Walking Warm-up

Spend three of your ten minutes on this exercise—one minute forward, one backward, and one sideways. Walk forward and backward across the pool in chest-deep water until you've become accustomed to the water temperature. Now walk sideways, first leading with your pain-free hip, then leading with the painful hip.

Exercise 2. Bouncing: Backward, Forward

Bouncing backward is easier than bouncing forward, so start backward. Face the side of the pool, slowly bend both knees, and lower yourself to a half-squat position. Gently straighten both legs at the same time and take a small jump backward. Immediately bend both knees again and smoothly continue bouncing backward across the pool. Now try bouncing forward.

Exercise 3. Bicycling

Brace yourself at the side of the pool or sit on a step. Bend your knees to begin kicking in a bicycling movement as shown in Photo 1.

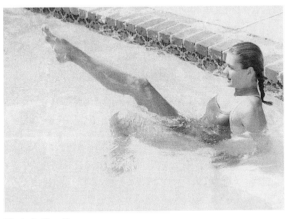

Photo 1. Bicycling.

Exercise 4. Hip Openers

Sit on a step to do this exercise or push your lower back against the side of the pool and brace yourself as shown in Photo 2. Open your legs wide apart as shown in Photo 3, then pull them back to the starting position. Continue opening and closing them, using equal force throughout both halves of the movement.

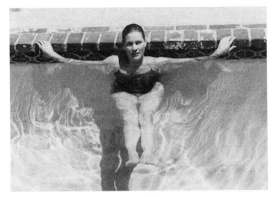

Photo 2. Hip openers, closed position.

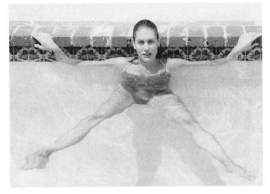

Photo 3. Hip openers, open position.

Exercise 5. Leg Swings

To protect your lower back, tighten your abdominal and gluteal muscles as you do this exercise.

Stand erect with your hand on the side of the pool for stability. Swing your left leg straight forward as shown in Photo 4, then swing it down and to the rear as shown in Photo 5. *If a full swing backward hurts your back, don't reach so far.* After thirty seconds, turn and perform leg swings with the other leg.

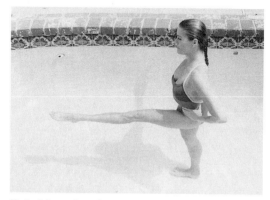

Photo 4. Leg swings, forward.

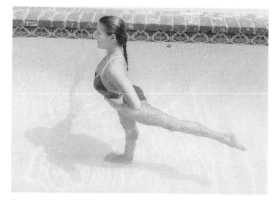

Photo 5. Leg swings, backward.

Listen to Your Body

As you position yourself for these exercises, you might feel the urge to move your leg or body in a way that isn't part of the program. That's your body talking to you: do what it tells you. For example, if you feel like pulling your knee toward your chest to loosen your back and buttocks, do it. Intuitive knowledge surfaces in the water, so pay attention to what you're feeling and what movements your body asks of you.

Exercise 6. External Rotation and Internal Rotation

If you've already had hip surgery, skip this exercise for now.

Stand on your right leg with your left knee bent and your thigh parallel to the surface of the water. For stability, tighten the muscles of your standing leg and buttock. Turn your knee outward to reach the position shown in Photo 6 (external rotation), then inward to the position shown in Photo 7 (internal rotation). Reach as far as you can in each direction. After thirty seconds, turn and repeat with the other leg.

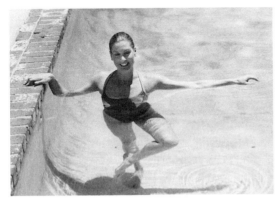
Photo 6. External rotation.

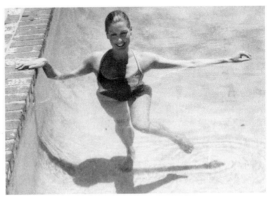
Photo 7. Internal rotation.

Exercise 7. Squats

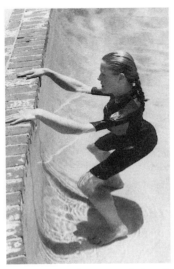

Face the side of the pool in chest-deep water with your feet parallel and shoulder-width apart. Grasp a gutter or the lip of the pool with both hands. Keep your back straight and slowly bend both knees until you've lowered your chin to the water as shown in Photo 8. Your heels will probably lift away from the pool bottom.

Photo 8. Squats (O'Neill wet suit shown).

Water Works!

Here's how water works: As soon as you step into the pool, you've eliminated the weight-bearing part of your problem. Once you've taken a "load" off your painful hip, you move it through its range of motion against the smooth, three-dimensional resistance of the water. Your hip gets stronger. Water is like a strategic missile that knows its target and continues to pursue it. No matter how you move in water, it works to strengthen the muscles surrounding your hip joint.

Exercise 8. Lateral Split

Grasp the side of the pool or an AquaTrend Pool Bar as shown in Photo 9. Gradually walk your feet away from each other, opening your legs to the side as far as you comfortably can. Breathe slowly and deeply as you hold this stretch for a minute.

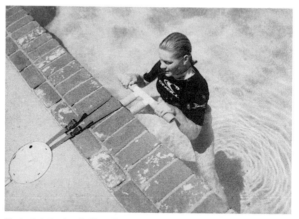

Photo 9. Lateral split (AquaTrend Pool Bar and O'Neill Thermo Shirt shown).

You'll probably discover that you don't want to get out of the pool after only ten minutes. It feels so good you'll want to return day after day.

Ten-Minute Land Program

When you return from the pool, find a carpeted space where you can comfortably lie on the floor for these exercises. Although Exercise 10 addresses both hips at the same time, the others require that you do one side, then repeat on the other. Therefore, we've allocated two minutes to each exercise, which includes the time you'll need to rest between exercises.

Exercise 9. Abductor Stretch

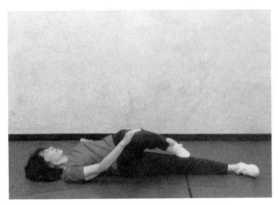

Photo 10. Abductor stretch.

Lie on your back with the knee of your uninvolved leg bent and your involved leg flat on the floor. Pull your uninvolved leg across your body as shown in Photo 10. Your opposite hand is out to the side for balance. Hold this stretch while you breathe deeply and slowly five times. Consciously relax with every exhalation. Come back to the starting position, then perform an abductor stretch on your involved side. Repeat on each side.

Exercise 10. Internal Rotator Stretch

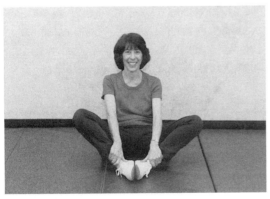

Photo 11. Internal rotator stretch.

Sit up with your spine erect and your knees bent to the sides. Put the soles of your feet together with your hands around your ankles as shown in Photo 11. Relax and breathe deeply at least five times while maintaining this position.

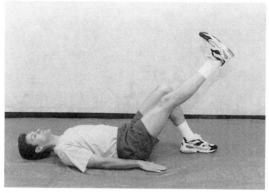

Photo 12. Straight leg raise.

Exercise 11. Straight Leg Raise

Lie on your back with the palms of your hands flat on the floor beside your hips. Your right leg is straight, your left leg is bent, and your left foot is on the floor. Keep your right knee straight as you lift it to the position shown in Photo 12, then return it to the floor. Do this eight times, then repeat on the other side.

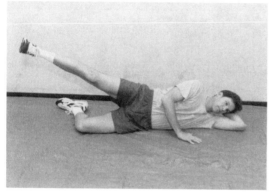

Photo 13. Abduction.

Exercise 12. Abduction

Lie on your side with your unaffected hip up, your body in a straight line. Lift your unaffected leg as high as you can, as shown in Photo 13, then slowly return it to the starting position. Do eight of these on each side.

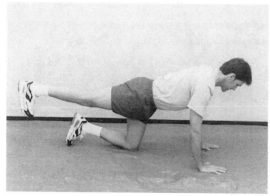

Photo 14. Extension.

Exercise 13. Extension

Assume a balanced position on your hands and knees. Then lift your right leg out behind you until your leg is parallel with the floor, as shown in Photo 14. Return to the starting position on your hands and knees. Do eight on each side.

After your ten minutes in water and ten minutes on land, you will probably feel your hip moving more smoothly and with a greater sense of ease. You have just discovered an important truth: Movement heals.

2

Healthy and Unhealthy Hips

Go to your freezer and take out two ice cubes. Wet them and rub them against each other. Feel how slippery they are. There is almost no friction as one glides across the surface of the other.

Next consider a healthy hip joint. The two surfaces of that joint are even more slippery than the ice cubes. As the hip bends, rotates, and straightens, the contact between the two halves of the joint is so delicate that the coefficient of friction—the amount that they rub together—is less than that of your two ice cubes.

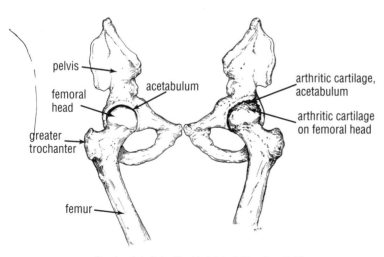

The hip is where the thigh bone (femur) attaches to the pelvis in a ball-and-socket joint. (See Drawing 1.) The upper end of the femur is shaped like a ball and forms the **femoral head.** That head rotates in a socket called the **acetabulum,** which is formed by the pelvic bones. The hip joint is extremely strong, and at the same time it is durable and offers great range of movement.

Drawing 1. Left, healthy hip joint; right, osteoarthritis.

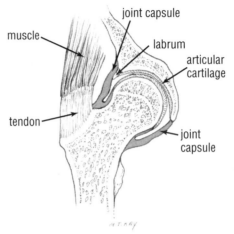

Drawing 2. Hip joint capsule with surrounding soft tissues.

The tough fibers and ligaments that encase the hip joint are called the **joint capsule.** These connective tissues envelop the joint and hold it together. (See Drawing 2.) Surrounding the joint are muscles and tendons that attach those muscles to the bone. Those muscles are located in the buttocks, the pelvis, and the thighs, and they control movement at the hip. **Bursal sacs** filled with fluids are situated in key spots around the hip and act as cushions to prevent friction and relieve pressure between moving parts. Running through the soft tissues around the hip are various sensory and motor nerves that carry impulses *to* the brain to create sensation and *from* the brain to the muscles to create voluntary movement.

In a healthy hip, the femoral head is covered with a layer of rubbery, gel-like tissue about one-eighth of an inch thick called **hyaline cartilage** or **articular cartilage.** The acetabulum is lined with this same articular cartilage. When the hip joint moves, the femoral head rotates in the acetabulum, but since articular cartilage has no nerve endings to transmit signals to the brain, you are not aware of movement between the two cartilage layers, and you don't feel any friction. Nor do you feel the constant trauma of weight bearing when you walk, run, or do any of your other physical activities. This miraculous cartilage that provides such elegance is like your permanent teeth: you get only one set.

Articular cartilage does not have a blood supply. Rather, it receives its nourishment from a flow of fluids. When the joint is at rest, the spongy material that comprises cartilage soaks up liquid, primarily synovial fluid. Then when you put pressure on that hip joint by taking a step, it squeezes the fluid out again. When you lift your leg to take another step, the fluid rushes back into the cartilage. The fluid moves in and out as your cartilage responds to the changing forces exerted on your hip joint.

The Muscles That Move the Hip

Muscles work in synchronized pairs: when one contracts, the opposing one relaxes. The muscles executing the actual movement are known as **agonists.** As the agonists contract, the opposing muscle group, the **antagonists,** must relax to allow movement to occur. For example, when you lift your leg forward, the hip flexors serve as the agonists to initiate the movement, while the opposing hip extensors, the antagonists, relax to allow movement to occur. Conversely, if you reach your leg backward, the muscles reverse roles: the extensors are the agonists, while the flexors are the antagonists.

The muscle pairs of the hip are the flexors/extensors (Drawings 3 and 4 on page 12), abductors/adductors (Drawings 5 and 6 on page 12), and internal rotators/external rotators.

External and internal rotators combine the muscles shown in Drawings 3, 4, 5, and 6. Photos 6 and 7 on page 5 show the actual movement of external and internal rotation.

The Negative Spiral: Loss of Hip Function

Once you start to feel pain or limited movement in your hip, a downward spiral begins. If you've been aware of your pain for a while but have taken no measures to combat your hip condition, you may have already entered this Negative Spiral, shown in Figure 1 on page 13. First you feel pain or limitation of movement, so you move your hip less often. You stop running, bicycling, and working out in the gym.

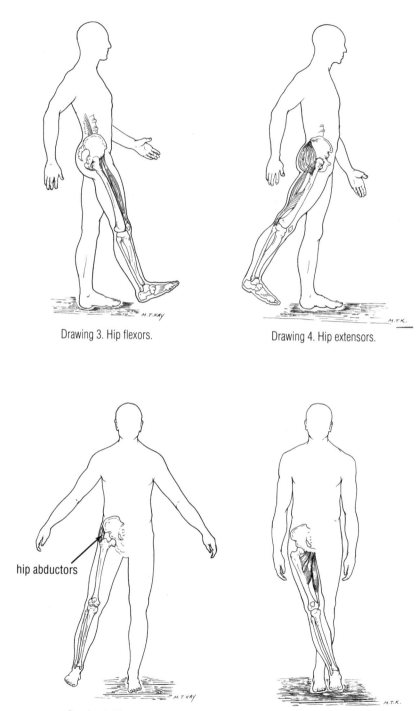

Drawing 3. Hip flexors.

Drawing 4. Hip extensors.

hip abductors

Drawing 5. Hip abductors.

Drawing 6. Hip adductors.

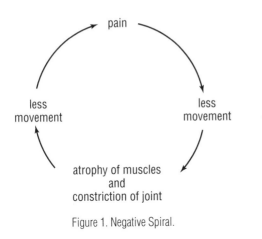

Figure 1. Negative Spiral.

You begin driving your car to places you used to walk to. As the pain continues, you may even find yourself not answering your phone because it seems too far away. Because you are no longer moving your hip joint, it isn't receiving the fluids and nourishment it requires, and it becomes further constricted and inflamed. The muscles begin shrinking, a process called **atrophy.** Once these muscles start feeling weak, you use them even less, and they atrophy even more. The tendons and capsule around the hip joint aren't being stretched to their usual length, and they begin to lose their elasticity. They become brittle and likely to split or break.

Here's an analogy that you can apply to your sore hip: Imagine you've broken your foot and doctors put it in a cast so the bones can heal. But they also confine the muscles and tendons of your calf. When the cast comes off weeks later, the X ray looks fine, but your leg is shriveled from disuse. Now you have aches and pains coming from the tissues that were immobilized. The tendons haven't moved, so they weren't lubricated and they lost flexibility. The muscles didn't contract, so they atrophied and lost strength. In the same way, if you stop moving your hip due to pain, you are virtually placing your hip in a cast, and the muscles and tendons around your hip will suffer the same fate as those around the broken foot.

It is indeed a Negative Spiral: lack of movement causes increased soft tissue involvement, which in turn causes more pain, so you move even less.

You want to turn this cycle around, and you can. You can bring the soft tissues back to health, which eliminates the secondary aches and pains.

If you've bought this book, you probably already have pain or limited motion in your hip joint. If you nodded with recognition while reading about the Negative Spiral, you may have already decreased your activity and begun noticing that your hip is getting worse. It's time to learn more about what is going wrong with your hip.

The Main Causes of Hip Problems

The six main causes of hip problems are:

Osteoarthritis
Posttraumatic arthritis
Rheumatoid arthritis
Hip dysplasia
Avascular necrosis
Soft-tissue injuries

Osteoarthritis

Osteoarthritis is the most common cause of hip problems. It affects millions of people worldwide, including more than fifty million Americans. Known as the "wear-and-tear" form of arthritis, it was formerly thought to be caused by excessive stress to the joints from high-impact activities, but more recent studies tell us that regular exercise does not predispose us to osteoarthritis. In fact, regular exercise can increase the functional capability of osteoarthritis patients.

Called OA for short, osteoarthritis appears in two distinct forms: primary and secondary. Primary OA is the most common and usually strikes the weight-bearing joints after the age of forty-five. We don't yet know the exact cause of primary OA, but obesity and family history are known to be risk factors. Secondary OA often appears before the age of forty and can usually be linked to a specific cause such as injury, the use of certain medications, or even joint infection or metabolic imbalances such as gout.

As we age, OA can dry out our crucial cartilage, deteriorating this protective cushion between the bones. As the disease progresses, the cartilage begins to grow brittle and to crack. Its surface may become pitted and uneven. There may even be "potholes" on the surface (see Drawing 1 on page 10). Although osteoarthritis begins in the articular cartilage and is primarily focused on the cartilage, it also affects other areas in and around the hip joint, including the muscles and tendons adjacent to the joint, the capsule surrounding the hip joint, and the **subchondral** bone at the ends of the bones just below the cartilage.

Symptoms of Arthritis

The classic early symptom of arthritis is that you know when it's going to rain. When the barometric pressure is changing quickly, you start to feel the deep, deep pain of arthritis. Other signs of arthritis specifically in the hip include pain when first standing up after sitting for a while, and loss of internal rotation, which means not being able to point your toe inward.

Your body has the ability to tell you that something is not quite right. Around an arthritic joint, your body might give you a clue with **tendinitis** (see page 21). Mysteriously, the pain is not always in the spot where the real problem is. In the very early changes of arthritis in the hip, don't be surprised if your knee isn't feeling just right or if you're having a groin muscle ache. That can be an early tip-off that something isn't right deep in the joint nearby.

The other types of hip problems are described below. If your symptoms don't fit into any of those categories, you probably have osteoarthritis.

Posttraumatic Osteoarthritis

Posttraumatic osteoarthritis is virtually the same thing as osteoarthritis except that it is caused by previous structural damage. The damage doesn't have to be in the hip, either. Trauma to an ankle or a knee that leads to a leg-length discrepancy can lead to arthritis of a hip. Injury to any weight-bearing joint—the lower back, the hip, knee, foot, or ankle—can cause eventual damage to adjacent joints. In fact, the injury doesn't even have to be on the same leg. A right knee injury could cause problems with a left hip. If you fractured your leg or even your ankle years ago, that may have altered your gait such that you became arthritic in your hip.

A former professional basketball player now in his sixties had knee surgery that left his knee unable to straighten completely. Several things began to happen over the next few years. The muscles surrounding the knee could no longer go through their full range of motion, so they began to atrophy (decrease in size) even though this athlete worked extensively in the pool and in the weight room. Since the knee couldn't straighten, that leg functioned as if it were shorter and caused him to limp. Next, this athlete began bending at the hip when he walked to accommodate the abnormal function of his knee. Thus he began using his hip joint abnormally, too. The hip joint was no longer going through *its* full range of motion, and the same deterioration process began, first of the muscles, then of the other soft tissues surrounding the hip, and finally of the joint itself. His hip became damaged not because of trauma to the hip but because of trauma to the knee.

This is probably the easiest of all the categories of hip problems to diagnose, unless of course you've forgotten about childhood or adolescent injuries that could be the cause of today's orthopedic problems. Complete the careful body history questionnaire in Chapter 3, and perhaps you'll find clues regarding your current hip condition.

Let's say you broke your hip as a child or a teenager. Doctors fixed it, but let's look at how it was "fixed." Picture yourself holding two billiard balls. Imagine throwing one onto a concrete floor and seeing it smash into pieces. Even if you used the best glue possible and managed to reconstruct the ball to a perfect orb, you would still see dozens of seams. Surgeons may have put your hip back together with plates and screws and whatever else it takes to reconstruct the normal anatomy, but even so, your body knows the difference. Years later, the irregularities in your anatomy begin to behave like very fine sandpaper; in the long run, they are enough to wear out the joint.

The symptoms of posttraumatic osteoarthritis are nearly the same as those of basic osteoarthritis. The only significant difference is that if surgery has taken place, pain could be coming from the hardware—the plates and screws that were used to reconstruct the hip or femur or pelvis. The tip of a piece of metal could be sticking into a muscle or other soft tissue, causing inflammation. In that case, removing the hardware could relieve your pain.

Rheumatoid Arthritis

Rheumatoid arthritis (RA) is an autoimmune disease in which the body's immune system attacks its own tissues. For whatever reason, a miscalculation or perhaps a defect in the DNA, the immune system falsely identifies its own tissues as foreign substances and begins to attack them as if they were a bacteria or other invader to be eliminated.

RA affects more than two million North Americans each year, the majority of whom are women. In fact, RA strikes women three times as often as it does men. In its mildest form, its symptoms include joint discomfort, but if it progresses to its most serious form, it can cause painfully deformed joints and even harm the body's organs. The onset of this disease is typically between the ages of twenty and forty, which means that women are usually affected during their childbearing years.

All joints are lined with a synovial membrane, which is a two-layer membrane, on a bed of fat, composed of cells that normally produce synovial fluid. **Synovial fluid** is a transparent alkaline fluid resembling egg white. It is found in joint cavities, tendon sheaths, and bursae. When working normally, this fluid lubricates and feeds cartilage surfaces. In RA, the synovial cells that line the joint leak a corrosive enzyme that acts like battery acid on the tissue it encounters. The enzyme's damage to the cartilage is devastating: in effect, it peels the cartilage away, making it thinner on the periphery of the joint. Imagine a scoop of ice cream sitting in an ice cream cone. The scoop of ice cream is the ball in the ball-and-socket joint. The damage from the corrosive enzyme occurs where the cone meets the ice cream, that juncture where the cartilage stops and the bone begins. These are **periarticular erosions.** (In Latin, *peri* means around, or the perimeter.) These periarticular erosions start on the line around the joint rather than at the dome of the cone, because that's where a large number of synovial cells are found. It's the synovium that destroys cartilage, so that's where the cartilage damage occurs first. As the erosion continues, it eats its way toward the top of the dome of the ice cream. A classic way of diagnosing RA is to see a reduction in total bone mass called **osteoporosis** showing up as washed-out-looking bone on a patient's X rays along with the defects and crevices where the cartilage stops and the regular bone begins—periarticular erosions.

Osteoporosis can also be caused by the medicine RA patients take. Or by disuse! If the pain of swollen and inflamed joints causes patients to cease their normal activities, they are no longer putting a load on their bones. That's a signal to the body that there's little stress on the bones, so the body starts to reabsorb more bone from the joints and the surrounding bones.

The bottom line with RA is that the joint lining is destroying the joint. All areas that have lubricating surfaces get involved: that means the tendons, ligaments, and cartilage are all affected. Often you'll see deformity taking place in the hands of RA patients. Where osteoarthritis causes a knobby type of knuckles called Heberden's nodes, RA patients will often get an angulation to their hands so that the fingers are turned to the outside. Their fingers, wrists, and hands can be irregularly shaped in many different ways. (The French artist Renoir was thought to have RA, because the hands that he painted, probably while looking at his own, showed these deformities in the works he painted in his later years.)

RA is probably passed down genetically, although some experts think it could be caused by a bacterial infection in the joints. Others say it might be triggered by a virus in people who are genetically susceptible.

Early symptoms of rheumatoid arthritis include joint swelling and pain with no history of trauma or infection. Later, rheumatoid nodules can form at the tips of the elbows and on the feet and knees. These fatty bumps are under the skin and can become debilitating if they cause the skin to break down. If other diagnoses have been ruled out for your hip problem, it may be the systemic disease RA.

Hip Dysplasia

Hip dysplasia is a congenital condition in which the hip socket develops abnormally over an entire lifetime. If the ball of the hip isn't inside the socket during the development of the fetus and infant, the two pieces of the hip don't have a chance to mold to each other. A **coxa magna,** or mushroom-shaped femoral head, develops, because the socket wasn't able to guide its growth into a smooth, round shape. On the socket side, what is supposed to be a nice round dome becomes a flatter surface because the ball wasn't there to force the round growth. Nearly always the deformity has led to a smaller, shallower socket. Only rarely does the deformity take the form of a larger socket than normal.

Hip dysplasia is something the hip develops from the fetal stage into early childhood, into early adulthood, and finally into adulthood.

This condition has its own clock: it can cause pain and limited function at any point in life. Dysplasia is usually diagnosed early in a person's life, so you probably already know if you have it.

Avascular Necrosis

The *a-* part of avascular necrosis means "without." *Vascular* means "blood supply." *Necrosis* means "death." So avascular necrosis, or AVN, is death to the bone because of an absent blood supply.

Think of your hip joint as a lake in the mountains. Some lakes have multiple streams that come down through the mountains to feed them, keeping the lakes full of water. Then consider a lake fed by only one stream. If you were to block one of the streams to a lake that has multiple streams feeding it, there wouldn't be much effect. It would still have what is known as **collateral circulation:** it's getting water from other sources, not just one. But if you were to block the stream to a lake that has only the one water source, the lake would go dry.

The hip joint, unlike other parts of your body, is like the lake that has only one stream feeding it. Drawing 7 shows the one major blood vessel into the hip joint. If that vessel is damaged in any way, your hip will lose its nourishing source to the bone, its blood supply, and it will

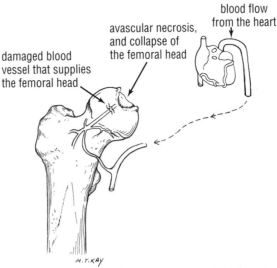

Drawing 7. Collapse of head of femur due to loss of blood supply.

die. Notice how the head of the femur has collapsed due to the death of the bone under the cartilage surface.

Trauma is a common cause of avascular necrosis of the hip. If you were in a sports accident or a car wreck and the femoral head or neck was broken, the blood vessel could have been torn, causing AVN. If you dislocated your hip, the ball went outside the socket and the blood vessels were stretched. The hip has to be put back into place within six to twelve hours. The longer the hip is out of position, the longer the blood vessels to the hip are being stretched and the greater the chance that the hip will die. With every hip dislocation, you're hoping the blood vessels were stretched, not torn, but you won't know for sure until some time goes by. You may see bone death right away or over time, but nearly always you'll see it within three months if it is going to occur.

Certain drugs can also cause AVN: steroids such as prednisone and cortisone are the main culprits. Most cases arise from long-term use of these medications, but there have been occasional cases that show that no matter how the drug got into your system—by intravenous injection or by mouth—it can cause serious negative side effects, including AVN.

In pharmacology we refer to drugs as being idiosyncratic in terms of people's responses to them. Two different people can take the same pill and can have similar or opposing reactions to it. One may take the drug with little or no side effects while the other may get stomach cramps and have allergic reactions. *Never take any medicine without your doctor's advice and without considering its possible effects.*

Alcoholism can be another cause of AVN. There are many theories as to why alcohol causes damage to the blood supply, but no one is exactly sure why. What is certain, however, is that the longer you remain an alcoholic, the greater your chance of developing avascular necrosis. Working for long periods as a scuba diver also has its dangers: if you contract the bends, a condition in which oxygen and nitrogen bubbles form in the bloodstream, you can cause damage to the hip's precious blood supply and develop AVN.

The symptoms of avascular necrosis usually include severe hip pain that comes on abruptly. A sudden absence of blood supply can cause an immediate, acute feeling of intense pain. Interestingly, the pain can be most intense in the beginning and decrease thereafter. (It's important to see your doctor right away.) Other symptoms include groin pain that goes down the front of your thigh and pain when rotating your leg side to side.

Soft-Tissue Injuries

The most common soft-tissue injuries are:

Tendinitis
Muscle strains
Bursitis
Capsulitis
Ligament strains
Muscle and capsule contractures

Tendinitis. Tendinitis is inflammation of the tendon that attaches muscles to bones. It feels like a sharp sticking pain whenever the muscle is contracted and can occur because of overuse or overstretching of a muscle. It can also be due to trauma: the tendon may be strained or partially torn. Hip-flexor tendons, up high at the front of the thigh, and the gluteal tendons where the buttocks meet the hamstrings are the two most common locations of tendinitis in the hip area. You can usually find the sore tendon by palpating (probing) the tissues with the fingers.

Muscle strains. Muscle strain is the tearing of muscle fibers. Strains can be mild or severe, depending on how many fibers are torn. The adductors and hamstrings are the most common muscles around the hip to be strained.

Bursitis. Bursitis, generally caused by trauma, impact, or overuse of the hip, is the inflammation of the **bursae,** or protective sacklike cushions in the joint. You may feel a sharp pain on the outside of your hip whether you are moving your hip or not.

Capsulitis. Capsulitis is an inflammation of the capsule that surrounds the hip joint. It creates a very deep hip pain that you feel whenever you move. Capsulitis can be due to trauma, overuse, or degenerative changes inside the joint.

Ligament strains. Deep in the hip, around the joint, are the ligaments that reinforce the integrity of the structure and keep it solidly together. It takes fairly severe trauma to the hip to damage those deep, ropelike ligaments, trauma of the caliber of a car accident or a bad fall.

Muscle and capsule contractures. A muscle contracture is a persistent shortening of a muscle; a capsule contracture is the constriction of a joint capsule. The result of either is deep, sharp, restrictive pain and limited movement of the hip. The most common limitation is a hip-flexor contracture in which the hip remains slightly bent at all times; further, the buttocks above the sore hip will lose strength and tone.

In spite of the many things that can go wrong with hips, there are steps you can take to alleviate the pain and limited function that accompany these various conditions. After you reach the right diagnosis in Chapter 3, you can immediately begin treatments suggested in Chapter 5, then start the pool and land programs in Chapters 7 and 9.

3

The Right Diagnosis: Doing Your Part

Times have changed. People no longer need to rely solely on their doctors for medical knowledge. Today we live in an information age when anyone can discover, with the click of a computer's mouse, the latest developments in the diagnosis and treatment of medical conditions. And because you are reading this book, you're now one of the many who are making an effort to understand their own hip problems.

Hip Help

To be your hip's best friend, keep up with the latest research on new hip treatments and check regularly the latest information I make available on my Web site: www.hiphelp.com.

—*Robert Klapper, M.D.*

A Written Physical History

A good way to continue delving for information is to prepare a physical history. Use the form that follows to trigger your thinking. Go over each item carefully, and as you do, you'll probably surprise yourself by remembering events of years ago. You may also think of details not included on the form. Write them down. Begin to keep track day by day of your pain: how often your hip hurts, what time of day it seems to hurt most, and what kinds of things you do that relieve the pain.

A caution: people often say that their hip pain "came out of nowhere." Such statements offer no help in a diagnosis. Better to think hard about the recent past, about a fall or other event that could have damaged 95 percent of one of the structures of your hip. No pain ensued at the time, but weeks or even months later, when the other 5 percent of that same portion of the hip was damaged by something as simple as bending to pick a flower, pain began. With such lag time between the inciting event and hip pain, your job becomes that of a detective. Dig back into the past. It's easy to forget a fall from a ladder or a slip off a curb if no pain resulted. Yet most of the injury could have been caused at that earlier time.

A final caution: don't overlook a remembered pain that was once acute but then vanished and never returned! To understand how this could have happened, consider an analogy: A woman starts a new gardening activity that strenuously uses her hands and develops a blister on her palm that causes acute pain. She gives the blister a few days to heal, then continues gardening off and on over the next months. The blister eventually turns into a callus, the pain completely deadened.

Remembering such a previous flare-up of hip pain can greatly help in diagnosing your condition.

Physical History

What is your hip problem?
    Pain ___
    Limping, but no pain ___
    Faulty gait or walking pattern ___
    Limited movement ___
What is the location of your pain? (Circle all that apply.)

	L = Left	R = Right	B = Both
Side of the hip	L	R	B
Lower back	L	R	B
Groin	L	R	B
Thigh	L	R	B
Knee	L	R	B
Foot	L	R	B

When did the pain start?
    After trauma ___
    After a heavy workout ___
    After a fall ___
    Gradual in onset with no specific beginning date ___
    Other, explain _____

_____

Have you had a problem with your hip(s) in the past?
    As a child ___
    Wore leg braces as a child ___
    As a teenager ___
    New problem ___
    Other, explain _____

_____

Is your hip problem associated with work or the exercises you're doing?

_____

_____

What relieves the pain? _____
What makes it worse? _____
What medications are you currently taking? (Please include aspirin, over-the-counter medications, birth control pills, etc.) _____

_____

(continued)

Have you taken any new medication(s) in the last year? _____

Have you had prior treatment, tests, or diagnoses on your hip(s)?
   In the past year ___
   Many years ago ___
   Please be specific _____

What have you done for the pain?
   Nothing yet ___
   Visiting doctor ___
   Taken anti-inflammatories (aspirin, Motrin, Advil) ___
   Changed fitness routine ___
   Ceased exercise program ___
   Using a cane ___
   Using crutches ___
   Using a wheelchair ___
Do you drink alcohol?
   Occasional social drinker ___
   Several drinks every evening ___
   Alcohol intake has gone down in the past year ___
   Alcohol intake has gone up in the past year ___
Has your environment changed in the past year?
   Started working ___
   Stopped working ___
   Changed jobs ___
   Moved to a new home ___
   House has more stairs ___
   Office has more stairs ___
Have you moved to a new climate?
   Moved from humid climate to dry ___
   Moved from dry climate to humid ___
Have you begun wearing new shoes? Explain. _____

Are you exercising on a different type of terrain (grass, dirt, asphalt)? _____

Have you had recent surgery or pain involving other parts of your body?

How is the rest of your health? _____
_____

Have you had recent weight changes?
  Loss of ___ pounds in the past ___ months
  Gain of ___ pounds in the past ___ months
  No change in weight ___
Has anything changed in your driving habits?
  New car ___
  Longer commute ___
  Shorter commute ___
Has anything changed in your sexual habits?
  Pain during sex ___
  Increased activity ___
  Decreased activity ___
Have you had a recent increase in travel?
  Increased air travel ___
  Increased car travel ___
  Increased train travel ___
Have your sleep patterns recently changed?
  Increased due to lack of energy ___
  Decreased due to pain ___
  Erratic due to intermittent pain ___
Do you scuba dive?
  Never ___
  Occasionally ___
  Regularly ___
  History of any long scuba dives or diving accidents ___
Have you changed your diet? If so, how? _____
_____
_____

Are you having trouble with the activities of daily living?
  Walking ___
  Going up and down stairs ___
  Getting in and out of the car ___
  Putting on and taking off shoes and socks ___
  Getting up and down from a sofa or chair ___
  Other, list _____
_____

The Home Self-Examination

Once you've completed your written history, sit facing a full-length mirror for a self-examination. Breathe comfortably and relax until you feel you are sitting as you normally would.

Notice whether both your feet are pointing straight forward or whether one or both of your feet are externally rotated (turned outward) further than usual. Look for a "Charlie Chaplin" foot placement, the opposite of pigeon-toed. If your right foot, for instance, is pointing toward the right rather than straight ahead, we would say your right leg is externally rotated. Perhaps both of your feet have pointed outward ever since you can remember. In this case, noticing external rotation may not be significant. But if you've never been aware of external rotation and now you see just one foot pointing outward, this becomes significant: it may be an early sign of arthritis in your hip. Even if you have no pain in your hip to indicate the beginning of a problem, this may be a silent signal that your hip no longer has its normal rotational capability and that the surrounding soft tissues are becoming affected.

Inspect the way your shoes are wearing. Your shoes are like the tires on your car; they can tell you if your alignment is off. So notice if there's a difference between one shoe and the other. Notice if you're wearing through your newest shoes faster and in a pattern different from your usual wear pattern. This subtle difference could be an early indicator of arthritic changes in your hip joint or problems with the soft tissues surrounding the joint.

Watch yourself in the mirror as you take off your shoes and socks. See if you're making abnormal movements. Is it difficult or impossible for you to bend your hips enough to reach your foot? Does your knee have to turn outward so you can remove your shoe? Are you "cheating" by using your other foot rather than bending down to remove your shoes or socks? If you find abnormalities in these movements, they could indicate restrictions of movement in your hip.

Assess your toenails. Do they look in need of care because you aren't able to bend enough at the hip to maintain hygiene and keep them clipped? This is another silent symptom of hip problems.

Wearing only your bathing suit or underwear, stand and look at yourself in a full-length mirror. Are you standing straight or are you leaning? Do you have most of your weight on one leg? A hip contracture (a soft-tissue condition) may have you standing most comfortably on one leg with the other one slightly bent. A leg-length discrepancy could have you leaning to one side.

Get dressed and go up and down some nearby stairs. Are you able to **reciprocate** the stairs; that is, are you able to put your right foot on one step, your left foot on the next step, and continue in that manner? Or are you putting your right foot on a step, then putting your left foot on the same step in order to advance? A healthy hip is able to reciprocate going both upstairs and downstairs. Losing the ability to reciprocate stairs is one of the first changes in your gait you'll notice if your hip is unhealthy.

The Home Exam with a Partner

You may be walking abnormally, but because you've been doing so for weeks or even months, you no longer notice. You may also have become accustomed to having slightly swollen ankles or knees, so ask someone whose judgment you trust to help with this portion of the exam; wear shorts to allow your partner to examine your knees and ankles.

Wearing athletic shoes, walk back and forth so that your partner can observe you from the front, the back, and the side. Your partner will be able to tell if you are limping. If you're lurching or swaying from side to side, you have what's called an **antalgic gait**—an abnormal walking pattern that is due to pain. More specifically, it's a **coxalgic gait,** meaning the abnormal gait is due to hip pain. When you put weight on the hip that hurts, your body automatically compensates and makes an effort to take the weight quickly off that leg. If your partner is seeing this coxalgic gait, but you have no hip pain, the abnormal movement is probably being caused by weak abductor muscles on the outside of your hip.

If your partner sees your head bobbing up and down as you walk, that probably means you have what is called a short-leg gait. One of your legs might be longer or shorter in length because of arthritis, because of a fracture, or because one leg was shorter at birth. If the thigh bone (the femur) was badly fractured, the leg may have shortened when the two ends of the bone were brought together to heal. In some hip dysplasia cases, the ball is no longer in the socket. Instead, it's functioning somewhere near the socket, above or below, and that, of course, changes the length of the leg.

One of your legs could be shorter because a scoliosis (curvature of the spine) is forcing your pelvis to rotate, creating a leg that functions as though it were short even if it isn't anatomically shorter. Nearly all humans have a slight leg-length discrepancy, but a half-inch difference or more is usually necessary before a short-leg gait can be seen.

Remove your shoes and socks. Ask your partner to check for any swelling in either of your ankles or knees. Since you can't see swelling in the hip because big muscles surround that area, you look instead for swelling of the nearby joints. If both knees and both ankles are swollen, that could be caused by a problem with your heart. If only one of the four joints inspected is swollen, that often indicates a problem within that specific joint or a blockage of the blood flow to that leg. If one entire leg seems swollen, that could reflect problems in that hip. The irony is that you won't see the swelling in the hip, the actual site of damage; you'll see it "downstream," in the joints and tissue below.

Seeking Help from a Doctor

Once you've completed the written history and the self-exam and taken time to consider your answers, you're prepared to help your doctor diagnose and treat your unhealthy hip; that is, if you've decided to consult a doctor. Your reason for doing so may be as hard to describe as your "sixth sense." Or your reasons may depend entirely on the strength and duration of your pain, the loss of sleep due to pain, the restriction of your daily activities because of the soreness of your hip joint, or the alteration of your gait—at some point along the continuum of hip symptoms you'll decide to seek relief by combining your knowledge with a doctor's!

Schedule an office visit with your doctor and get an X ray.

Take along your written history for discussion during your initial office visit. For the moment, let me be your doctor. In the following items I've summarized the possible implications of your history.

Symptoms

How long have you had hip problems? Weeks? Months? Did the problem start suddenly or come on gradually? Is the pain associated with an acute event, an accident or injury, or has it been a slowly progressive problem? The location of the pain and the length of time it has existed will help in making a correct diagnosis.

Exacerbating Factors

When you've been sitting in a chair or lying in bed, do you feel a sharp pain in the groin or hip area when you stand and take your first steps? This is called **starting pain** and is considered **pathognomonic** to hip problems. Pathognomonic symptoms are the equivalent of a bull's-eye, the real signal that indeed you have a problem in your hip and not elsewhere.

Picture an auto mechanic in a small-town gas station. As you drive your car in, it's making a noise, and from across the garage the mechanic says, "It's your intake manifold, and spark plug number four needs to be changed." He hears in the way the car is idling what's wrong. The sound is pathognomonic to him. That's what starting pain is to hip problems.

Does your favorite workout or sport make your hip sore? Does the pain go away when you cut back on your recreational activities? You may have to choose your sports and workouts with more consideration for your hip.

Do you have hip pain after walking a certain length of time? When you sit down, does the pain go away? Answers to these questions will tell whether this is a circulatory or neurological problem. If your hip pain worsens as you walk but goes away completely when you sit down, that can indicate a circulatory problem. If, however, the pain in your hip and legs gets worse as you walk but it does not go away when you sit to rest, that may indicate a neurological condition such as a herniated disk or a pinched nerve.

Medications

Discuss with your doctor the medications and supplements you are currently taking: prescription drugs, aspirin and other over-the-counter pain relievers, hormone replacement, wellness supplements, amino acids, calcium, vitamin C, multivitamins, and birth control pills. Are you having side effects? Do you know which medicine or supplement is causing which effect? Have you taken any prednisone, oral cortisone, or other corticosteroids that may have *caused* your hip problem? Your dermatologist may have given you steroids for an outbreak of poison oak. Your eye doctor might have given you oral steroids for chronic conjunctivitis or other eye conditions. All this information is vital.

Deep joint destruction that erodes the cartilage and leaves the bone exposed can cause nerve pain. This kind of pain can't be relieved except by narcotics (codeine, for example), which mask all pain. If taking an over-the-counter anti-inflammatory can reduce some of the pain in your hip joint, that's a good sign that such severe destruction hasn't yet occurred; thus you might be a candidate for conservative treatment.

Prior Treatment

Have you seen another doctor or therapist for this hip condition? Have you had previous therapy, tests, or diagnoses? Have you had previous hip surgery or fractures? Did you have hip problems in childhood?

If you had surgery in childhood and an infection developed in any of the bones near your hip, that would be important to know, even if the infection was treated successfully. That infection may have destroyed some of the bone or the growth plate at the end of the bone, destruction that can lead to problems later on. If you have a poor recollection of your childhood, talk to your parents, siblings, or other relatives. If any of them have memories of your having had surgery or wearing a brace as a child, you owe it to yourself to get an X ray. Then you will know the status of your hip.

In the more recent past, you may have seen various doctors or therapists for your ongoing hip problem. The solution to one problem in your body in the past may now be the cause of your current hip problem. You need to assemble all the previous information you have gathered about your hip to give to your current doctor so you won't have to start the process all over again. Do your best to understand the conclusions other doctors have reached in order to summarize them during your conversation with your new doctor.

Sleep Pattern

Does hip pain keep you awake at night?

Because 40 percent of your body weight goes through the hip joint as you roll around in bed, a sore hip will wake people more often than any other joint. Such sleep deprivation is usually the end stage of the progression of hip problems: once hip pain starts affecting sleep, people who were reluctant to contact a doctor will now do so.

Functional Assessment

How well are you functioning in your daily life in spite of the problems you're having with your hip? Can you walk up and down stairs? Can you get in and out of a car? Do you need a cane to move smoothly throughout the day?

I watch my patients move around the office so I can have a glimpse of what their daily hip life is like. I watch how quickly or slowly they move, how they take their shoes off, how they get up from the chair. Do they grimace in pain as they stand up? I watch these things not because patients might be hiding something from me, but because I can sometimes see more in their movements than they can see themselves. They've made lifestyle changes, adaptations of movement that they no longer notice.

The Doctor's Physical Exam

Following this conference on your written history, ask your doctor to examine your entire body. Here is the way I examine my patients; I begin with gait.

Gait

I ask patients to walk down the hall so I can see how fast they move. I watch to see if they're limiting or shortening their steps or if they're leaning to one side. I notice if one foot is turned out or if both are. If the patient is limping, it's for one or more of these reasons: leg-length discrepancy, pain, or weakness of the abductor muscles.

Leg Length

Have you ever had a fracture of any of the bones of the leg or hip? Does one hemline of your pants appear longer than the other?

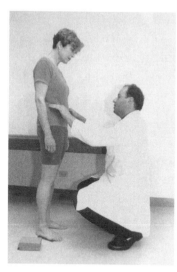

Photo 15. Measuring a leg-length discrepancy with blocks.

To measure leg length, I face the patient, who is standing barefoot in front of me. I place my hands on the top of her iliac crests (the top of the pelvis), as shown in Photo 15. My hands should be at the same level. If one is higher than the other, I have the patient step on blocks or lifts of differing heights until her hips are at the same height. If, when she stands on a quarter-inch block, her hips are level, she has a quarter-inch leg-length discrepancy. If there's more than a half-inch difference between the length of the two legs, I ask the patient to wear a lift in the shoe of the shorter leg in order to create better balance. If the discrepancy is less than half an inch, I tell the patient *not* to use lifts. If they aren't really needed, lifts can create back problems and hip problems. In my opinion, your body is better off without shoe lifts to cope with slight differences.

Examination of the Knees

As the patient lies on the exam table, I examine one knee and then the other. I assess the ligament integrity, range of motion, and the tracking mechanism (how well the kneecap rides within the groove of the femur). I check for a grinding sensation called **crepitus.** If the patient feels pain in either knee, we try to find its specific location. The most important thing is to discover if the pain is along the joint line of the knee. I ask the patient to bend her knees to a 90-degree angle, then I feel the kneecap. I feel the outline of it; then I feel the bottom portion of the kneecap, which roughly corresponds to the joint line. If there's tenderness in that area, this patient may have a problem with the shock-absorbing cartilage (**meniscus**) inside the knee joint. The meniscus could be torn or there could be early arthritic changes starting inside the knee joint. Pain, swelling, and limited movement in knees can also be caused by compensating for poor-gait mechanics caused by a sore hip.

It's extremely unusual for patients who have bad knees to be feeling pain in their hips. What often happens, however, is that patients tell me they have knee problems when, in fact, the problem is really coming from their hips. They feel pain down the front of the thigh that's emanating from the hip. Here's my theory on why this happens: The big muscles that run down the front of the thigh and into the kneecap are called the **quadriceps** muscles. *Quad* means four in Latin, and there are four muscles in the quadriceps group. One of the most powerful members of the quadriceps group is the rectus femoris. It is the most "superficial," meaning it is the closest to the surface. Drawing 8 shows that it has two heads, or two attachment sites. The first head is attached to the pelvis, but there's a deeper anchoring site for the second head, called the "reflected head." It attaches close to the front of

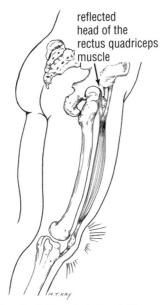

reflected
head of the
rectus quadriceps
muscle

Drawing 8. The reflected head of the rectus femoris can cause knee pain.

the hip joint capsule. If there's some heat or pain in the joint, it can sometimes radiate down the whole rectus femoris muscle, because one of the muscle's origin sites is sitting on an inflamed area. This means that patients who have an inflamed hip joint capsule often feel deep pain down the fronts of their thighs and are misled into thinking they have a knee problem instead of a hip problem.

Range of Motion of the Hips

The hip is capable of flexion, extension, rotation, abduction, and adduction. During our examination we assess all these planes of motion in order to determine whether there are any restrictions.

Flexion and extension. To evaluate the flexion of a patient's hip, I ask her to pull both knees into her chest. Normally one knee will be pulled closer to the chest than the other because the sore hip can't bend as well. I ask the patient to pull the knee on the healthier leg as close to the chest as possible and look at the amount of flexion that's

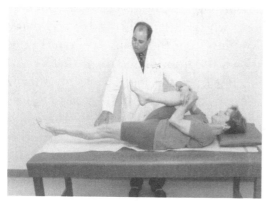

Photo 16. Hip flexion contracture.

possible. Then we compare that to the painful side. To check extension, I have the patient continue holding one leg and lower the other leg straight onto the table. If the leg doesn't go all the way down, as shown in Photo 16, the patient has a hip flexion contracture, which means that her hip is being held in a slightly flexed position by the soft tissues surrounding the hip. Either the muscles or the joint capsule are constricted and won't allow the hip to extend fully onto the table.

Here's how this constriction happens: When your hip joint doesn't move well through its entire range of motion, the muscles around it are no longer being stretched to their full movement. The affected muscles become fixed in their shortened state and are called muscle contractures.

Rotation. First we look at the healthier hip's internal and external rotation to establish the norm. Then we repeat the measurements on the painful hip. I test for external rotation by seeing how far your knee can fall to the outside: 0 degrees if your knee is facing straight up and can't turn at all to the side; 90 degrees if your knee can move so your thigh is parallel with the table. The average person has external rotation somewhere between 40 and 70 degrees.

Next we turn the leg in the other direction. The knee turns in and the foot angles outward, forcing the hip into internal rotation. The norm is different for each of us, but we want to see *some* internal rotation. We expect to see at least 10 to 20 degrees; 30 degrees would be a lot. This is a significant test, because internal rotation is usually the first movement to elicit pain in patients with an arthritic hip.

Abduction and adduction. When you **abduct** your leg, you move it directly to the side. To test for abduction, I pull the patient's leg wide to the side.

When you **adduct** your leg, you are bringing your leg back to or across the midline of your body. I put my hand on one of the bony prominences of the pelvis to feel whether the whole pelvis is rocking with the movement. I want to feel for myself whether the patient is getting movement because the hip is functioning or because the lower back and pelvis are moving. I want to see if there's any lack of hip-joint function.

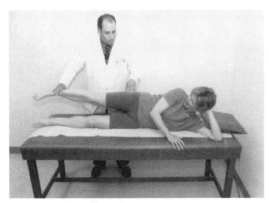

Photo 17. Test for bursitis.

Bursitis

The patient lies on her side on the exam table with the sore hip pointing toward the ceiling. We make sure the hips and knees are straight. Then I ask the patient to lift her whole leg as shown in Photo 17. She resists while I push down on the leg. If she has a single, sharp, discrete pain on the side of her hip while she's trying to resist me, we may have found a hip bursitis.

Ankles

I look at the ankles to assess them for swelling. Swelling could mean that a problem in the hip is disrupting the normal blood flow to and from the ankle. My other major concern is that the swelling might be indicative of a systemic problem such as lupus, rheumatoid arthritis, or a heart problem.

Neurological Exam

The human body has two kinds of nerves: sensory and motor. The sensory nerves transmit sensations from the body to the brain so you know what your body is feeling. The motor nerves transmit your intention to move from the brain to the muscles, causing movement. I test both sets of nerves. First, I test the foot's ability to register light touch and deep touch. I brush a piece of paper on the patient's foot to see if she feels it. If she doesn't, I could be picking up an early indication of diabetes.

A different set of nerve fibers register light touch and deep touch, so I test both. For deep touch, I apply pressure with my fingers on the top of the foot and ask the patient if she can feel it. Then I repeat the procedure on the bottom of the foot. I also check to see if the patient has sensation in the tips of her toes. After I've checked the sensory nerves, I test the motor nerves. I'll ask the patient to pull her foot upward and resist me as I try to push the foot down. Then I'll ask her to do the opposite movement, as though she were pushing down on a gas pedal. Again, I'll provide resistance and lift up against the force. If one leg is working well and the other isn't, we can probably assume nerve problems rather than muscular weakness.

Additional Tests

You may need additional tests for diagnosing your hip condition— blood tests or a lidocaine injection test. A blood test detects rheumatoid arthritis; a lidocaine injection test assures your doctor that a pinched nerve in your back is not causing radiating pain in your hip.

Most hospitals have a radiologist who is able to give the lidocaine test. Here's how it works: a machine called a fluoroscan provides X-ray guidance so that a needle can go directly into a hip joint to inject the numbing medicine lidocaine. If all pain goes away for four to six hours, we have confirmation that the cause of the problem is all in the hip, not in the back. If only 70 percent of the pain goes away, we conclude that 70 percent of the problem is in the hip and 30 percent must be coming from somewhere else.

More commonly used in diagnosing hip conditions are X rays, CT scans, and MRIs, which are discussed in the next chapter.

4

X Rays, CT Scans, and MRIs

Objective tests are the universal language of medicine. I could be in China and unable to converse with another doctor, but as soon as we put up the X rays, we would both be able to see what was happening in a hip joint. Similarly, once you learn the basics of looking at your X ray, CT scan, or MRI, you will begin to understand knowledge that is shared universally. In this chapter, I hope to give you the means to explain your hip complaints more clearly to your doctor and better understand his or her diagnosis.

Figure 2 shows a pelvic X ray. The patient's left hip (on the right) is normal, while his right hip (on the left) is unhealthy. First, let's look at the healthy side. Notice the ball-and-socket joint and the space between the two sides of the joint. Notice the whiteness (the density) of the bone. You'll return to this X ray several times as you read this chapter.

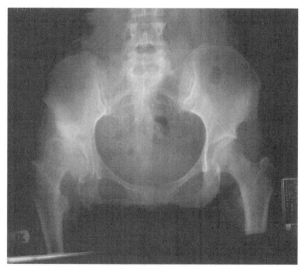

Figure 2. A pelvic X ray. On the right is a normal hip. Notice the smoothly curving surface on both the ball side and the socket side of the joint. The dark space between those two surfaces is cartilage. On the left is a hip with osteoarthritis. Notice the rough surfaces and that the cartilage is virtually gone—there's no longer a cushion for this joint.

In the classic teachings of medical school, there are subjective complaints of the patient, and there are objective findings, such as this X ray. The subjective complaints are things you tell your doctor about where you hurt, how badly you hurt, and how frequently. Although this information is crucial to helping your doctor reach a diagnosis, it has no real substance. But an X ray is something real, an objective finding you can actually see. So is a CT scan and an MRI. All three tests offer different kinds of information.

A **radiologist** is a medical doctor who has been certified as a specialist in interpreting X rays. **Orthopedists** and other physicians often consult with a radiologist for interpretation of the more complicated findings that appear on X rays. It takes years of training and experience to be able to read an X ray, CT scan, or MRI, so our goal isn't to make you a radiologist, only to demystify a complicated aspect of medicine. This knowledge can have a powerful effect on your body. For instance, scientific experiments routinely use **placebos** to test the effectiveness of drugs. The placebo is merely a sugar or salt pill, but if the person taking it believes it will cure him, many times he gets well. Just as placebos can improve a person's health simply through a belief that the pill is helping, real knowledge can help you visualize your hip problem, understand your options for treatment, and assume responsibility for healing.

If your X rays are taken in the doctor's office, they'll be developed in only a few minutes, and you and your doctor can look at them together. If they are taken at a hospital or at a radiology center, make the extra effort to pick them up yourself and take them with you to your doctor. It's important for you to look at your X rays with your doctor, not to settle for the radiologist's report.

I enjoy looking at X rays with my patients and seeing a lightbulb turn on in a patient's mind as the learning process unfolds. I get lucky when only one hip is having problems, because then I can say, "Here's a normal hip. This is why. And here's your hip that's bothering you. This is why it's abnormal."

If you might be pregnant, you should not have an X ray, CT scan, or MRI done. Before you have any of these tests, you'll be asked a series of questions to ensure your safety.

X Rays

X rays use electromagnetic radiation to penetrate solids and act upon photographic plates. The films that result give doctors a look at parts of the body that have density, such as calcium. Bones have calcium, so we see them on X rays, which are an indispensable tool in the orthopedic examination of a patient, exposing a fracture, dislocation, or other pathologic changes in hips.

Let's suppose you have a normal hip and a problematic hip. When you look at the X ray of the normal hip, you'll see a space between the ball and the socket of the hip joint. (See Figure 2, page 41.) That's where the end of the ball and the end of the socket meet, but on the X ray they're not touching each other. The space between them isn't air, it's the cartilage at the ends of our bones, but because cartilage doesn't have calcium, it doesn't show up on the X ray. When you see that space on an X ray, you can conclude there's a healthy cartilage space between the ball and the socket. The joint is normal. When you look at the abnormal hip and see the ball getting closer to the socket, that means a loss of joint space, a loss of cartilage, which means arthritis.

You also might see **spurs**—calcified outcroppings on either side of the joint. My opinion is that these spurs are the body's attempt to stabilize the joint when it becomes wobbly from cartilage loss. But spurs actually turn into part of the problem, because they are rough growths within the joint where there should be only smooth surfaces. Sometimes pieces of these spurs will break off and become **loose bodies,** or loose fragments inside the joint.

Sclerosis is a hardening of the bone. It's the opposite of osteoporosis. Osteoporosis—fragile bones—shows up on an X ray as washed-out bones, while sclerosis shows up as a denser, whiter-looking bone. As a joint becomes arthritic and begins to have problems functioning smoothly, it no longer shares the weight of the body equally on all its surfaces. The weight bearing becomes concentrated in certain spots of the joint, and those areas become denser: the X ray will show more sclerosis—a denser look to the bone there. Particularly, you'll see sclerosis in avascular necrosis. Without a healthy blood supply, the bone collapses like a sponge and becomes dense as it squashes down.

When you have an X ray, you'll be asked to take a breath and hold it so that you won't inadvertently move. Then you'll hear a buzz and that will be it. There will be no discomfort or sensation.

CT Scans

In the phrase CT scan, or CAT scan, the letters stand for computerized axial tomography. It is a three-dimensional X ray that shows all sides of the area under examination.

To understand the difference between an X ray and a CT scan, imagine that I have a ten-inch-long candle standing upright in a candlestick holder and that the wick is filled with calcium. If I take an X ray of that candle, the wax will disappear and the only thing that will show up is the line of the wick running vertically. Now, if I decide I need a CT scan of that candle, the photograph I get of the wick won't be lengthwise, but will instead be a slice right through the candle, and I'll be viewing the wick as if from above. I'll see it sitting like a doughnut hole with the wax as the invisible doughnut all around it. Now I can see the front, back, right, and left side of the wick, not just the vertical length of it. There will be a series of "slices" showing up in the pictures, so we can search for the problem. We will be able to see, for instance, that the wick isn't perfectly round at a certain spot, that it's indented on the right side and bulges out a little on the left side at a specific level. Or maybe the wick isn't as thick at one level as it is everywhere else. Then, to identify the location, I look at a localizer reference grid, which will tell me that the first photograph corresponds to the four-inch height level of the candle and the second photograph corresponds to the eight-inch height level.

The CT scan can take as many slices as are necessary. The radiologist can request ten slices in a ten-inch candle, or he can request thirty. (If, for instance, the radiologist is worried that a tumor might be growing in the wick, he can specify thinner cuts, which will provide more pictures and more information.)

An X ray tells us what the wick looks like from only one side, top to bottom, but the CT scan gives us a three-dimensional look from above at the entire circumference of the wick—front, back, left, and right—in the multiple places where it has been sliced.

Think of the socket side of your hip joint as a dome like the United States Capitol building. If the dome is deformed, I want to see what the front, the top, the back, and the sides of the dome look like. An X ray would give me a view of only the front of the dome, but the CT scan will give me the full picture, from every possible angle.

For the CT scan, you'll go into a room with a scanner and lie on a narrow platform. The platform slides into a doughnut-shaped tube that's about two feet deep. Most of your body will be outside the tube except for the portion that is being scanned. The platform will move you through the tube, stopping at specific intervals for each scan. The person taking your scan will be in the control room watching you through a glass window and speaking to you through a microphone. You'll be able to talk to the technician if you're uncomfortable or concerned about anything. Although thirty minutes is usually allotted for the scan, the actual scanning time is approximately fifteen minutes. During that time, you'll need to lie still. You won't feel anything, but you'll hear a whirring sound as the computer moves the X ray machine around your body. Most patients are relatively comfortable during the procedure.

MRIs

Unlike CT scans, magnetic resonance imaging (MRI) does not use X rays, but magnetism and radio waves. The powerful magnet requires certain precautions. If you have a pacemaker, you shouldn't have an MRI done, because the magnet could interfere with the pacemaker's function. If you've had brain surgery, you'll need to show documentation that metal clips weren't placed inside your brain. If you have tattooed eyeliner, the metal in the tattoo will cause the magnet to tug on your eyelids. This may be mildly painful, so you may want to put an ice pack on your eyes afterward. Other metals in your body such as rods around the spine or a hip implant tend not to be magnetic and therefore won't cause problems. You may feel local warming in those areas, but nothing of significance. You'll be asked to remove your keys, watch, hairpins, bra, and jewelry (rings excepted). If you opt to leave your earrings in place, you might feel a mild annoyance as they are pulled on by the magnet.

Make sure you don't have credit cards in your pocket, because the magnetic strips will be wiped clean.

Unlike X rays and CT scans, the MRI allows us to see both the bones and the soft tissues of the body. This means we can see swelling, bruising, and inflammation, the same type of inflammation, for example, that occurs inside the joint at the beginning stages of arthritis. You'll see fluid inside the joint and inflammation of the synovial lining. You won't see either of those things on an X ray. Bursitis will show up in the area of the bursa as fluid just below the skin. If a herniated disk is the source of your hip pain, you'll be able to see the bulging disk pressing on the nerve that is responsible for sensation and movement in the hip joint. An MRI offers a "sliced" view of the body as seen from above (like the CT scan) as well as side and angled views.

Sometimes an MRI gives us too much information. For instance, if I have to develop a surgical plan to reconstruct a patient's hip, I want the clear, crisp lines of an X ray to help me understand the geometry and the architecture, not the nebulous lines with all the information

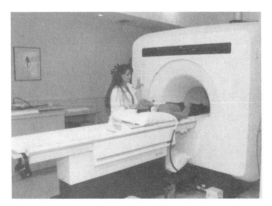

Photo 18. Entering an MRI machine. The patient is wearing headphones and a microphone.

an MRI gives me. The X ray lets me focus on the structure without anything else clouding my vision.

To have an MRI of your hip, you'll go into a room and see a large doughnut-shaped machine. The doughnut hole is a narrow tube more than six feet long at its center. You'll lie flat on your back on a padded, moveable platform that's about as wide as a stretcher, with your feet pointed toward the tube (Photo 18). Your feet will be taped together to keep your hips in the correct anatomical position. Your entire body, including your head, will slide inside the tube. The smaller you are, the more comfortable you'll be. A woman five feet five inches tall who weighs 125 pounds will experience the tube as being almost roomy, while another woman of the same height who weighs 175 pounds might have only a few inches on all sides of her body. The weight limitation for most MRIs is 300 pounds, because a body that size, unless it belongs to someone seven feet tall, would simply be too large in girth to fit into the tube.

For some patients, going into the MRI tube can be a claustrophobic experience. If you find it so, the radiologist can administer a sedative to calm you but not put you to sleep. Some radiologists use valium given orally or by injection. Injections, because they work instantly, are more predictable and controllable than pills. If you opt to use such conscious sedation, a clip will be placed on one of your fingers to monitor your pulse and oxygenation levels so that you won't be overmedicated.

If you truly think you could not withstand the MRI's confinement, take the time to search for an open-air MRI scanner, which will be easier on you emotionally; however, the quality of the pictures tends to be not as good. This technology will improve soon, but for now, the best pictures with the most information come from MRIs done in closed tubes.

Making the MRI More Comfortable

You might want to shop around for a more comfortable experience than a standard MRI unit. Some of them have these amenities: earphones so you can listen to music to drown out the jackhammer sounds of the magnet; a microphone so you can talk to the technician in the control console; a fan that blows air through the tube, giving the comforting sensation of standing in a breeze; or lights inside so you won't feel stranded in the dark. You might even want to look for an MRI that has accompanying virtual reality glasses. With these you can view a relaxing scene—a waterfall or the ocean—while the minutes pass inside.

Figure 3. X ray of rheumatoid arthritis. On the left is a normal hip. On the right you can see an absolute loss of delineation between a ball and a socket. It almost appears as though the femur has been fused to the pelvis. This shows the destruction caused by RA as it has eaten away the cartilage between the ball and the socket of the hip joint.

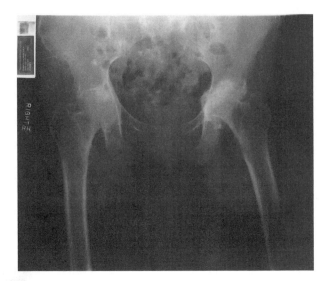

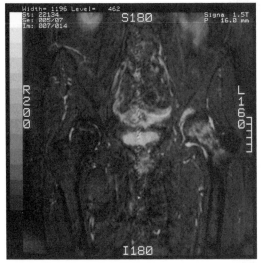

Figure 4. MRI of avascular necrosis. On the right, notice the white marrow of the bone and the integrity of the sphere, which is the ball of the ball and socket joint. On the left, notice the blackness within the ball, which represents the death to the marrow and the lack of blood supply to the ball.

Figure 5. X ray of post-traumatic osteoarthritis. Twenty years ago this man was in a car accident that required a series of screws in his femur and pelvis for the reconstruction of his right hip (on the reader's left). Severe damage to the cartilage meant eventual deterioration of the joint, but he was able to heal enough to provide enough bone stock so that now, at fifty, this man had implant surgery, the screws were removed, and he now has an X ray that mimics the usual one seen after implant surgery on page 148. He has complete range of motion and a pain-free hip.

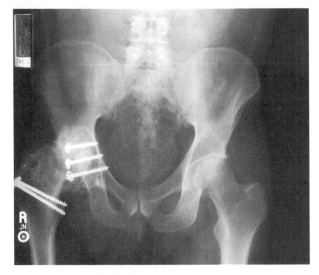

Keep Your Own X Rays

The world of medicine is changing. So are insurance plans, Medicare, and health maintenance organizations (HMOs). Doctors come in and out of your life. The only constant is *you*. You need to do everything in your power to keep your current X rays in your possession and carry them with you when you visit various doctors. If anyone refuses to release your X ray, respectfully ask for a copy. At the very least, you'll want to have a copy of your pelvis X ray like the ones in this chapter. Keep all your X rays together in the large envelopes they come in, and store them in a cool, dark place. Put them flat on top of everything else in a closet or another location where you won't lose them.

Here's an illustration of how important your X rays can be. Recently I saw two patients who were told they needed hip surgery. They each came to me for a second opinion. One patient was in his late seventies, the other in her early eighties. These patients had had implant surgery over twenty years ago. I could see on each X ray that the plastic was wearing out on the socket side of the joint. However, neither was having much pain. Still, they were told they had to have a revision of their hip surgery.

Both of those patients brought along old X rays. I compared their X rays from four or five years before with the new ones and saw no difference. The wear on the plastic had not increased in the past five years. Neither patient was complaining of pain, so I told them both they don't need surgery but to hang onto their X rays and that we'd keep an eye on their condition over time. I wouldn't have been able to make that recommendation without their old X rays.

5

The Right Treatment: Doing Your Part

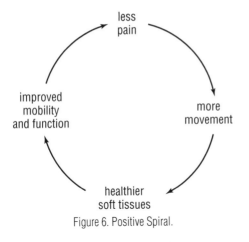

Figure 6. Positive Spiral.

Now, with commitment to treatment, you'll enter the Positive Spiral to hip health: less pain leads to more movement, which leads to healthier soft tissues, which leads to improved mobility and function, and so on (see Figure 6). Begin by choosing among these conservative treatments that will allow you to enter the Positive Spiral at the point of LESS PAIN.

Getting Unstuck

I've gathered anecdotal information over the past twenty-five years from coaching injured athletes in water and on land, and I've reached an interesting conclusion: if a person's pain starts shifting location slightly or the symptoms begin changing, the injury is trying to heal. The body is innately programmed to heal; that's what it does best. When pain is "stuck," unchanging, it seems the healing process is stuck as well. You need to do something to get "unstuck." All of the treatments described in this chapter can start the process.

—Lynda Huey

Reduce High-Impact Activities

Reduce the duration of your everyday high-impact activities by climbing fewer stairs, carrying fewer heavy packages, avoiding standing in long lines, doing less taxing yardwork, or walking shorter distances. In addition, modify your sports life: Replace high-impact activities with (in this order) water workouts, bicycling, and running on a treadmill or other soft surface such as grass or sand. If you are a former athlete who can't bear to give up your favorite sport completely, you should use one of the recommended activities for daily fitness and save your sport for soul-satisfying special occasions.

Wear Impact-Absorbing Shoes

The harder your shoes, the more impact you are transmitting to all of your weight-bearing joints, including your hip. That translates to more trauma to the articular cartilage surfaces and more erosion. Wear the highly cushioned athletic shoes made for runners. That may not be realistic all the time given the demands and dress codes of your workplace, but wear them whenever you can.

Take Anti-Inflammatories

Phone your doctor to ask if you can begin taking nonprescription anti-inflammatories such as aspirin, Advil, Motrin, or Aleve. Your doctor knows the medicines you're already taking. He will tell you how these new drugs might interact with your prescription drugs. Commit to using the anti-inflammatories only for a month or two, knowing you'll soon wean yourself from such pills and depend on the natural drugs your body manufactures when you exercise.

Lose Weight

Your hip is the largest of your weight-bearing joints. Every time you take a step, you load your hip with more than three times your body weight, so if you weigh 150 pounds, your hip has to support over 450 pounds with each step! Every pound you gain means more than three pounds of pressure placed on your hip with each step. Conversely, if

Losing Weight

There's no mystery about losing weight. You have to increase your exercise and cut down on your eating. Most people can't manage this very well alone, so get whatever help you need. Join an exercise program or hire a personal trainer to motivate you to work out consistently. Choose one of the many weight-loss organizations that are available. Create an exercise/food management program that you're comfortable with so you'll stick with it and really take off some fat. Your hip is at risk, so get serious. If you've tried to lose weight many times and failed, consult with your internist or a nutritionist.

you were to lose ten pounds, you would eliminate thirty pounds of pressure that your hip must bear. *Now is the time to lose weight by dieting and starting a low-impact exercise program.*

Cortisone Injections

It is well known in the medical community that injecting cortisone into a joint damages the surfaces of the vital articular cartilages in that joint. Yes, cortisone is a miraculous anti-inflammatory that knocks out pain and swelling (sometimes temporarily, sometimes forever), but it may damage working surfaces of the joint and can leave behind, to linger forever in your joint, the gritty, powdery substance found in some cortisone preparations. Repeated injections into a joint literally "spoil" that joint. Doctors know that, but we look at the trade-off.

    Yes, I've injected cortisone into a hip on exceptional occasions: a desperate patient, going to Europe, couldn't exchange his plane tickets; a distraught mother with debilitating pain wanted to walk down the aisle at her daughter's wedding. In both cases I made sure the patient understood the risk.

—*Robert Klapper, M.D.*

Glucosamine and Chondroitin Sulfates

These two supplements are showing great promise in treating early stages of osteoarthritis. The authors of *The Arthritis Cure*, Jason Theodosakis, M.D., M.S., M.P.H., Brenda Adderly, M.H.A., and Barry Fox, M.D., suggest that glucosamine sulfate helps preserve healthy cartilage cells by retaining shock-absorbing water, while chondroitin sulfate protects the cartilage from destructive enzymes.

Modalities

When doctors or physical therapists speak of using a modality, they are referring to the application of a therapeutic agent. These therapeutic agents can be anything from ice to heat to electrotherapy. They are all modalities, and they help arouse the body's natural healing forces while decreasing pain and swelling. While they can make you feel better, they are strictly an adjunct to the exercises that are the true heart of your program. Modalities can be a temporary solution to pain; improved strength and flexibility are the long-term solution.

Ice

Ice is the most underrecognized of all painkillers. It needs no prescription, is easy to apply and quick to begin working—and it's free. Applying ice to your sore hip reduces blood flow, slows nerve conduction, and elevates your pain threshold. Because it cuts your pain, it reduces your need for pain medication. Keep in mind that ice treats only the tissues closest to the skin—it works well in reducing muscular pain, tendinitis, and bursitis, but it won't reduce pain or swelling deep inside your hip joint.

Fill a large plastic freezer bag with ice cubes and place it on the part of your hip where you feel pain. If your skin is particularly sensitive, put a thin cloth between the ice bag and your skin. Leave the ice bag in place for ten to fifteen minutes, but check your skin under the ice several times to make sure your skin hasn't been burned by the ice. When you

A Free Miracle

Ice is the closest you can come to a free miracle. It can knock out pain and speed the healing of many injuries. Look at ice as a quiet but powerful cure. I swear by it and advise all those I work with to ice after leaving the pool.

—Lynda Huey

remove the ice, wrap a dry towel around the cold skin. You will feel the area start to thaw. If your hip hurts in more than one place, move the ice to another sore spot for another ten to fifteen minutes.

If you become a devoted fan of ice, you'll want to give your hip an ice massage. Fill a Styrofoam cup with water and put it in the freezer. Once frozen, peel down the Styrofoam until about an inch of ice is exposed. What's left of the cup becomes a "handle" for this ice massage device. Begin making circular or back-and-forth motions with the ice cup on the sore areas of your hip. When your skin turns pink and feels numb, wrap your hip in a dry towel.

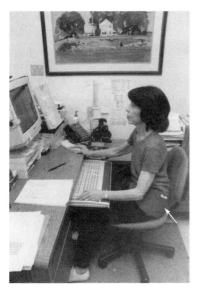

Photo 19. Continuing daily activities while icing the hip with ICE/HEAT (indicated by arrow).

For convenience and adjustable compression as well as complete mobility, the reusable ICE/HEAT by Tru-Fit can be used instead of ice bags. ICE/HEAT consists of a freezable gel pack that fits into an insulated soft fabric encasement with stretchy Velcro straps to wrap around your body. The straps stay snugly around you, holding the gel pack in the most desirable position over your hip, buttocks, or groin. With the ICE/HEAT firmly in place, you can continue your daily activities at home or at work with none of the mess of ice bags. (See Photo 19.) The gel pack can also go into the microwave and be heated to offer contrast treatments discussed next.

Contrast Ice and Heat

Ice decreases cell metabolism and increases tissue stiffness. Heat increases cell metabolism and decreases tissue stiffness. Both ice and heat decrease pain. Use ice as the *only* treatment for the first forty-eight hours if you have a sudden or **acute** injury to the hip. If the hip problem is considered **chronic,** both ice and heat can be used. Apply heat. Follow it immediately with ice. Go back and forth several times: heat, ice, heat, ice—this alternation is called *contrast ice and heat.* Heat causes **vasodilation,** an increase of blood supply to the area, then ice brings about **vasoconstriction,** a decrease in the blood supply. These contrast treatments confuse the body by bombarding it with stimulants that are opposites. The confusion causes an escalated response and a tremendous amount of circulation and healing to the area.

At home, use a heating pad or place your ICE/HEAT gel pack in the microwave for one minute to create a hot pack. In fifteen minutes, switch to ten minutes of ice. As the ice treatment begins, you may feel a deepening of the pain, an aching from the cold. Then as the numbing occurs, virtually all deep pain is gone. When the heat is applied again, the cold tissues go through a "thawing" sensation that most people find pleasurable. Finish your contrast treatment with ten minutes of ice. Hot showers, baths, hot tubs, and cold pools are also appropriate contrast treatments for pain management. In the hot tub, sit in a position that allows the jet stream to flow directly toward the sore area of your hip.

Physical Therapy

Physical therapists offer various treatments, including massage therapy, ultrasound, and therapeutic exercise. (See Chapters 8 and 9 for more details about physical therapy.)

Massage therapy. By kneading, elongating, and gently manipulating soft tissues beyond their restrictions, the therapist relieves muscle spasms, softens tight and inflamed tendons, increases blood flow, and generally aids in restoring health and function to the hip. When the therapist's hands are exerting pressure to the tissues, you will often feel increased pain, but as soon as the pressure is released, your tissues will feel more mobile and less painful.

Ultrasound. Therapeutic ultrasound mechanically vibrates tissues at an extremely high frequency. This micromassage raises the tissue's temperature, which improves circulation, resulting in increased cellular metabolism, thus accelerating the healing process. Ultrasound is applied to the skin through a water-based gel. Medications can be added to the gel so that the ultrasound drives the medicine through the skin into the underlying tissues. When ultrasound is used in this way, it is called **phonophoresis.**

Therapeutic exercise. Chapter 6 introduces you to the pool program in Chapter 7. Chapter 8 explains some of the physical principles behind the stretching and strengthening program in Chapter 9.

Chiropractic

Chiropractors perform manipulations that can free joint and nerve restrictions that cause hip pain. Some chiropractors offer the same ultrasound treatments done by physical therapists.

Acupuncture

Acupuncture has been a standard medical practice for thousands of years in China, and it has endured for a reason—it obviously helps heal. Acupuncturists use needles to relieve pain and stimulate the body's natural healing systems.

Yoga

Yoga offers a series of sustained stretches that you can do without outside assistance. (In Chapter 8 you'll see sustained stretches done to a hip patient by a physical therapist.) If you have limited range of motion in your hip but your X rays show no mechanical reason for the lack of movement, consider yoga and stretching as a way to relieve your pain and gain flexibility. Yoga postures are held for several minutes each, and the slow, deep breathing that accompanies these positions reduces muscular tension and pain. As you relax deeply into each sustained stretch, your hip joint gradually opens, giving you more movement in every plane.

> **Yoga**
>
> Choose your yoga class carefully. You'll find a vast array of classes, but many of these have diluted yoga's original intent of slow stretches combined with deep breathing and meditation: they've become westernized "workouts." Search for a traditional yoga class that most likely has its roots in India. You want a class that focuses on stretching, not sweating. Your intent is to relieve pain, not stress an already troubled hip joint.

Aquatic Therapy

Exercising in water—aquatic therapy—can be the best of all pain-reducing treatments. It naturally increases circulation, releases endorphins (the body's painkillers), and stimulates the body's healing mechanisms.

Further, exercising in water is the gentlest, safest way to increase flexibility, increase strength, and gain endurance—in other words, the best way to regain movement, mobility, and function. A more detailed description of the unparalleled qualities of water appears in Chapter 6.

When you followed the pool program described in Chapter 1, you used water's buoyancy to move your hip through its entire *current* range of motion. It may have moved more easily in some planes of motion than in others, for example, forward and backward more easily than out to the side. You may have found pain as you stretched your legs wide apart. You gained information about your painful hip that you wrote into your physical history and talked over with your doctor. The longer, more comprehensive pool program in Chapter 7 will show you how to progress along the Positive Spiral.

6

Getting Started in the Pool

When your hip joint becomes disabled, you can't move well, at least not on land; but in water you're able to move in a natural manner. Water's magic lies in its buoyant support for the body, its resistance to bodily movement, the pressure it exerts on a submerged body, its ability to reduce pain, and its relaxing and refreshing feel.

Buoyancy is the upward thrust exerted by water on a body that is totally or partially immersed in it. It lifts the body and provides a feeling of weightlessness. If you stand in waist-deep water, 50 percent of your body weight is supported by the water. If you move to chest-deep water, 70 percent of your body weight is lifted from your weight-bearing joints. In neck-deep water, 90 percent of your body's weight is eliminated, and if you put on a flotation device and move to deep water, you are virtually weightless. By thus neutralizing gravity's downward force on your hips, you are able to exercise in greater comfort and perform movements that are not possible on land.

The resistance the water supplies to the body during movement is considered the workload, just as a stack of weights in the gym is the workload during a weight-training session. Water offers isokinetic resistance, meaning that it matches the resistance you give it. As hard as you push, it pushes back with equal force. This is a safe and efficient way to strengthen even the sorest hip, because you'll never meet more resistance than you can handle, since the resistance always equals the force you applied. (In Chapter 8 you'll learn about Cybex and Biodex machines that cost thousands of dollars. They duplicate on land the kind of resistance that water offers naturally.)

The amount of resistance the body encounters in water is directly proportional to the speed of the movement. For example, if you move your leg at a slow speed through the water, you feel a gentle resistance. Then, if you move your leg exactly twice as fast through the water, you will encounter exactly twice the resistance. The water automatically adapts to your demands and becomes an instantly variable training gym. You can do more or less work, move faster or slower, on any given exercise, depending upon what you feel you need.

The hydrostatic pressure exerted by the water on the submerged surfaces of the body is proportional to the depth of submersion. In other words, the deeper you are in the water, the greater the hydrostatic pressure. Think of the water as working on your entire body, like a support stocking works to keep swelling out of your feet, ankles, and calves. Water provides support for unstable joints, it helps venous blood return to the heart, and it relieves swelling, especially in the arms and legs. As you move, the massaging effect of the water on your body helps loosen and lengthen tight muscles while the hydrostatic pressure helps flush out waste products such as lactic acid from tired tissues.

The sensation of water on your skin acts as a counterirritant to reduce your pain. Because nerve impulses stimulated by water on your skin are faster than those stimulated by pain, the skin impulses literally beat the pain impulses to the brain for recognition. The end result is reduced pain.

Exercising in water promotes relaxation. The water encourages you to perform gentle, rhythmic motions, which can reduce muscular tension and improve limited range of movement. Further, the mental and emotional stress that comes with pain and impaired physical capability is immediately reduced when you begin movement in water. You perceive less pain and feel more capable, so your body and mind begin to relax.

Regaining Motion

Hydrostatic pressure may have another interesting benefit. It may be that the stimulus of the water against your skin enhances the communication between the brain, the muscles, and the joint. That extra communication link can help guide you safely through your pool program as you regain motion that has left your movement vocabulary.

Benefits of Water Exercise

Exercising in water offers unique benefits to a hip wellness program. You'll feel them as soon as you enter the pool, but first take the time to understand the basic principles at work.

Balanced Strength in Muscle Pairs

Back-and-forth movements of the arms, legs, and trunk are possible only because muscles work in synchronized pairs—when one contracts, the opposing one relaxes. These muscle pairs maintain a specific ratio of strength to each other. If that ratio is thrown out of balance by injury or arthritis, or by training only one of the muscles in a pair, inefficiency and the potential for injury result. Therefore it is extremely important to exercise both muscles of each antagonistic pair: quadriceps/hamstrings, abductors/adductors, and so forth.

Although you could forget to strengthen one half of a muscle pair on land, that can't happen in the water. Every exercise in water forces you to work both halves of each muscle pair. For every push forward against water's resistance, you must pull backward to the starting position. For every swing upward, you must swing downward. When you exercise in water, symmetry is built in.

Movement Possible Only in Water

In addition to forward and backward and side-to-side movements, the hip joint is capable of a unique circular motion called **circumduction.** On land there is virtually no way to resist the hip joint evenly as it moves through its complete range of circular movement. In water, however, when your hip performs circumduction, it encounters equal resistance from the water throughout the entire movement, thus gaining maximum strength through its complete range of motion. (See Leg Circles, Exercise 22, page 102.)

Aerobic and Anaerobic Fitness

Aerobic fitness allows for moderate, continuous endurance exercise such as hiking for six miles without stop. Anaerobic fitness is necessary for strenuous bursts of speed and explosive power such as running up a flight of stairs. Both aerobic and anaerobic fitness are vital to a well-conditioned person.

If you suffer from hip pain, it may be impossible for you even to think of performing such activities on land. Continuous aerobic exercise that consists of weight-bearing movements can aggravate your hip through overuse and make your muscles feel heavy. Anaerobic training, by its nature, is powerful, explosive movement that could further damage a deteriorating hip.

In water, however, sore hips are often capable of walking, running, and even jumping so that aerobic work is achieved effortlessly and anaerobic work sneaks in almost painlessly. You can feel a sense of great strength against the water's resistance, yet because of the greatly reduced gravitational pull, you should be able to finish the workout feeling fresh and having encountered little pain.

Improved Flexibility

Although stretching is a peaceful and soothing activity for most people on land, for some hip patients it produces discomfort and strain. If you avoid most stretches due to hip pain, you will benefit greatly from stretching in water, where comfort and relaxation are built in. You'll find that you can assume positions to perform stretches in the water that you couldn't possibly assume on land. Further, enjoying stretching means you'll do it more often, for longer periods of time, and with more regularity. That adds up to faster progress.

Increased Range of Motion

The water's buoyancy offers you a somewhat unexpected gift. You'll find that your hip can move forward, backward, and in complete circles much more easily than it ever would be able to on land. This increased range of motion is something you don't have to force. Water's buoyancy will naturally lift your leg higher, wider, and further each session without your having to think about it.

Improved Balance

In water you are constantly using your abdominal and back muscles as well as your arms and legs to maintain erect body alignment and balance. Increased strength in these muscles, plus focus on a constantly changing balance point in water, will lead to improved balance on land that will carry over into your daily activities.

Increased Coordination

When you walk or run on land, your right arm and left leg move at the same time: this is called cross-crawl patterning. In water, many people become disoriented regarding the opposition of their limbs. It may take some practice and attention to master this, but the result will be well worth the effort, for water training increases overall coordination by emphasizing cross-crawl patterning, which is the basis of *all* human coordination.

Improved Gait

Because of ongoing hip pain, you may have developed an uneven walking pattern or gait, and you may have lost strength in the abductor muscles that stabilize your pelvis. The gait-training exercises starting on page 87 will help you create new habit patterns that are symmetrical and balanced at the same time that they force new strength into the weak muscles.

Correcting Habits

Abnormal gait can be caused by weak muscles or bad habits. For instance, your knees may cross the midline of your body when you do Exercise 1, Deep-Water Running (page 76), either because you've developed that bad habit or because your abductor muscles are weak and can't control the movement, allowing your knees to collapse inward instead of moving straight forward.

Use your mind's discipline to correct the weakness and your faulty gait at the same time: every time you force your knees to lift straight forward instead of following the path of least resistance across your body, you strengthen the muscles and you correct the habit as well. As the abductors grow strong from being used, rather than favored, you'll make the proper movement not only out of your new habit but also because the muscles are now balanced from exercising correctly.

A Sense of Well-being

What an amazing change in attitude you can experience as soon as you enter the water! Stress washes away. You'll take a deep breath and notice your shoulders and neck have relaxed. You'll feel better simply for having submerged in water.

The Equipment You'll Need

It isn't necessary to invest in expensive equipment to begin participating in a pool program. All you need to get started is a pool, a bathing suit, and a flotation device. Other equipment can be added as your improving strength seeks challenge and variety. (A list of all products and manufacturers appearing in the text can be found in the appendix.)

Your Suit

Men should choose a comfortable pair of trunks. Be sure they have a tie-string to make them snug around the waist so they will stay up when you jump or bounce. Women should wear one-piece workout suits, not sun-bathing fashion suits or bikinis. You will be performing a variety of exercises and won't want to be distracted from your form and technique by having to hold your suit in place.

Flotation Devices

Every flotation belt or vest has its advantages. Consider the details given here as they relate to your own body density and structure.

The AquaJogger. The AquaJogger was the first buoyancy belt manufactured for deep-water exercise. Like the flotation belts that were developed later, the AquaJogger allows for full range of motion of both arms and both legs in all body positions, from vertical to horizontal. The AquaJogger is held around the waist by an adjustable, elastic belt with a quick-release buckle. Its wide design in the back provides stability and support for the lower back. The AquaJogger Pro (extra buoyancy) model is recommended for those with low body-fat percentages. The economic AquaJogger Basic is made out of stiffer foam but does the same job for those who are watching their budgets.

Hydro-Tone Belt. This black ensolite foam belt with vinyl coating places buoyancy evenly around the waist. The Hydro-Tone Belt is held in place by two narrow canvas straps with quick-release buckles. This is the most buoyant of all the belts and should be considered for use by dancers, athletes, and other "sinkers" who require extra buoyancy.

Wet Belt. This foam belt offers good support for the lower back and is easily adjustable on both sides of its removable strap. The narrow belt at the front makes it comfortable during all stretches and exercises.

H.A.N. model Wet Belt. This one-size-fits-all strip belt distributes buoyancy evenly around the body. The cloth-covered foam comes in two strips, which are held together with easy Velcro fastenings that make the belt adjustable at the front *and* at the back. This belt works best with people who float easily.

Speedo Aquatic Exercise Belt. This teal-colored belt provides extra buoyancy for those with low body-fat percentages. Its narrow construction makes it comfortable during all stretches and exercises. The clasps are a combination of quick-release buckle and adjustable strap with Velcro to keep the loose end of the strap under control. This belt is made of closed-cell foam and covered with vinyl. It dries quickly, making it a good choice for traveling.

Wet Vest and Wet Vest II. These buoyant vests were the first flotation pieces specifically designed for deep-water running and walking. They are the only flotation devices that will float you in a "heads up" position if you are motionless. (The belts all tend to tip you forward unless you make gentle, correcting movements.) The Wet Vest goes on like a standard vest. A "beaver tail" attaches through the legs to keep the vest down and in place against the water's buoyancy. The Wet Vest II goes on over the head like a bib, then connects with the beaver tail and side-wrapping panels. The Wet Vest II is cut lower under the arms to prevent chafing and allows for more variation in body size, so several people of various sizes can use the same vest.

Support Equipment

When you first learn deep-water exercises, you may have trouble finding your center of balance. A few simple pieces of equipment can make the job of learning these new exercises easier by offering buoyant support.

Hydro-Fit Hand Buoys. One floating Hand Buoy in each hand can help you find stability in deep water if that is difficult at first. The buoys allow you to use your upper body strength to help maintain vertical alignment. The Hand Buoys can be held in front of the body, or held with one on each side of the body.

Hydro-Fit Swim/Therapy Bar. Some people like two small Hand Buoys while others prefer one long therapy bar to help them maintain their balance in deep water. These tools make it easier to learn new deep-water exercises.

Resistance Equipment

Resistance equipment forces the body to move more water with each exercise. It is the equivalent of lifting more weight in the gym and is very effective strength training. *Resistance equipment should not be added to your program until your hip has been pain-free for several weeks.*

Hydra-Flow Water Weights. Contrary to their name, these are not actually weights, but rather cuffs made of vinyl mesh that strap around your shins. They are filled with polystyrene beads that create both lift and resistance during all leg movements. The slight buoyancy offered by the cuffs helps increase range of motion in your hips. These relatively new pieces provide a much-needed transition from using *no* resistance equipment during leg exercises to the powerful resistance offered by the Hydro-Tone Boots and the forceful buoyancy of the Hydro-Fit Cuffs.

Hydro-Tone Boots. Using the Hydro-Tone boots during your lower body exercises allows you to approximate closely a weight-training workout. These yellow plastic pieces snap on around your lower leg and foot and interact with the water along all planes of movement. They deliver smooth three-dimensional resistance throughout all of your leg movements. Anyone with a shoe size of over 9 for men and

10 for women should buy the standard model with what's called a TPU foot strap. If your shoe size is smaller than that, get the easier-to-put-on model that comes with a scuba sock attachment and a back zipper.

Hydro-Fit Buoyancy and Resistance Cuffs. These durable, multifunctional cuffs can strap onto the ankles, wrists, waist, or upper arms. In a hip program they will most commonly be used around the ankle to offer buoyancy and resistance during lower extremity exercises. If you're summoning courage to try the deep-water exercises, you might first try the cuffs around your upper arms. When used that way, they are similar to the "water wings" children use. They provide flotation and a solid sense of security.

Helpful Equipment

Some additional equipment will add comfort and stability to your pool session. As your pool program becomes a way of life, you may want to invest in these pieces as well.

Aquatrend Pool Exercise Bar. This new piece of equipment is the solution for home pool owners who have no gutter or bars to hold during kicking and stretching exercises. It is made of plastic tubing and covered with lightweight foam for a comfortable grip. The Aquatrend Pool Exercise Bar easily slips into the skimmer box and clips firmly into place with adjustable canvas straps and quick-release buckles.

Speedo Surfwalkers. Water shoes can protect your feet and provide traction at the pool, beach, or boat. If you tend to blister easily, or if your pool bottom is slippery, wear pool shoes. If you have diabetes, rheumatoid arthritis, or if you've had hip implant surgery, you should *always* wear shoes, not only in the pool but going to and from the pool as well. You want to take every precaution not to step on anything and get an infection.

The Waterpower Workout Tether. This well-constructed tether has a sturdy nylon waistband that is attached to a length of latex tubing. It fits snugly over your flotation device and attaches from your waist to the side of the pool. If you're having trouble establishing good deep-water running and walking form, the tether will offer you stability and significantly improve your posture. In shallow water, the tether lets you run at top speed without slipping or moving around the pool.

You might worry, especially after hip surgery, that a stray swimmer won't notice you and bump into you. You can make your location known to all swimmers by tethering yourself in one spot and staying there while you do your deep-water exercises.

Clothing to Keep You Warm

When you first begin the hip pool program, you may be moving quite slowly. If your pool is the standard 82 to 84 degrees, you'll probably find yourself getting cold and starting to shiver within twenty minutes. In order to be comfortable in cool water, consider investing in one of the following items specifically designed to keep you warm. Use the O'Neill Thermo Shirt or Thin Skin if you're feeling slightly chilled, but use a wet suit if you're downright cold.

O'Neill Thermo Shirt. Made of 90 percent polyolefin and 10 percent spandex, these stretchy pullover shirts offer protection from the sun's ultraviolet rays as well as insulation against cool water. They come in long-sleeved and short-sleeved models as well as various weights and colors.

O'Neill Thin Skin. This pullover shirt is made of half-millimeter-thick neoprene with a low crewneck collar and an elastic waist. Choose from a variety of colors in either short-sleeved or long-sleeved models.

O'Neill Wet Suits. Wet suits are generally made of neoprene and come in many lengths and thicknesses. For most pools you'll find that a "spring" suit is best, one that is designed to cover your body to the elbows and to the knees. Most suits easily zip up the back with the aid of a long nylon string. You should be quite comfortable in a two-millimeter spring suit even if the pool temperature is only 80 degrees.

The Pool

You may have one in your back yard or at your gym. You may have to search to find one that will provide you with the depth of water you need and the appropriate temperature. The pool you use for hip rehabilitation should have a shallow end with chest-deep water for your specific height. For example, if you are five feet three inches, chest-deep water is approximately three feet nine inches. If you are six feet tall, chest-deep water is closer to four feet six inches. You ideally want to have a relatively flat or unslanted pool bottom so you can walk across the pool at that correct depth. Besides chest-deep water, you'll also need water that is so deep your feet won't touch the bottom of the pool. For most people, this means you need water at least six feet deep.

When you first begin your program, you might be moving quite slowly. Water temperatures of 88 to 90 degrees will be most comfortable for you. As you progress and begin moving more strenuously, you'll feel comfortable in water that is 84 to 86 degrees in temperature. Unfortunately most people don't have access to the perfect pool or control of the ideal water temperature, so if you have to decide between the two, choose a pool that has the proper depth of water for you even if the water is cooler than you'd like. You can always make yourself warmer with additional protective clothing as mentioned above.

Nowadays nearly every community has a pool that can be used for a small fee. Your local college, YMCA, YWCA, YMHA, or recreation department are your best bets for finding inexpensive access to pools. Health club membership fees can be expensive, but they usually have plush facilities, including a sauna, steam room, or jacuzzi. Hotels may offer pool memberships to the neighborhood.

Check your potential pool's schedule. Make sure there is a recreational swim time during which you can use the pool without interference from lap-swimmers, children, or divers. Ideally, the pool you choose for your water training should be no more than ten to fifteen minutes from your home or workplace. The locker room should be clean, inviting, and comfortable. If your "home" pool is easily accessible, and if you are comfortable in its surroundings, you'll go more often than if it's unattractive or a long drive away. Next, find a backup pool for emergency use. You'd hate to find an unexpected "Closed" sign on your main pool and have to miss your aquatic therapy for a week or two just because you hadn't located an alternate pool.

Private Compact Pools

With the recent explosion in water exercise and aquatic therapy, new options have been developed for providing the main ingredient: water.

Small pools are now available and being used in therapy clinics, hospitals, and athletic training rooms. Even private homes can house a small indoor pool such as the HydroWorx and SwimEx for year-round exercise and therapy. They are modular in construction so they can go through most doorways to be installed in preexisting rooms.

HydroWorx. The HydroWorx is made of stainless steel and has adjustable handrails that can be placed in various configurations around or across the pool. You can run or swim against the current produced by three large jets on the front wall. This pool is twelve feet long and eight feet wide. The movable floor can be lowered from the existing floor surface to as low as six feet. Patients on crutches or even in wheelchairs can be easily placed on the unit, as shown in Photo 20, then the floor can be slowly lowered into the water. With the railings in place, the patient can easily stand and begin doing gait training, as shown in Photo 21. The entire floor is a treadmill with speeds varying from a crawl to 10 miles per hour. The floor is cushioned and designed to give the sensation of walking or running on wet sand. When the floor is lowered further, the patient can put on a flotation belt or vest and do deep-water exercises.

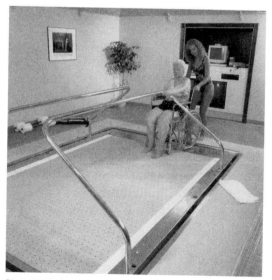

Photo 20. HydroWorx with the pool bottom level with the floor for easy access.

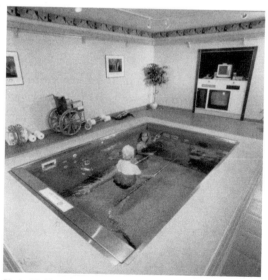

Photo 21. HydroWorx with the pool bottom lowered for gait training.

Notice that the patient can observe her own walking technique on the monitor. Two cameras are placed in front of underwater windows at the front and the side to send pictures to the monitor. Those images can be recorded for future viewing on the attached VCR.

SwimEx. The SwimEx pools are eighteen feet long and eight feet wide. They vary in depth according to the model. All models are equipped with a paddlewheel propulsion system that creates a broad flow of water that is fully adjustable with over forty different speeds—

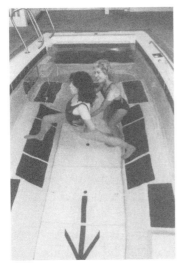

Photo 22. Stretching in a SwimEx pool.

from 0 to 6.5 miles per hour. You can swim or run in place against this variable current. The original SwimEx (400T) is forty-two inches deep and has a totally flat floor with a nonskid surface. The 500T model is fifty inches deep and has ten-inch floor inserts available to bring the water depth to forty inches. The Multi-depth 600T model is five feet deep with a twelve-inch insert that raises the water depth to four feet, thus accommodating people of various heights. It also features a running platform and eight work stations, including angled surfaces around the bottom perimeter, making it easy to perform various stretches and exercises. (See Photo 22.) The most advanced model, the 700T, adds a seventy-two-inch deep-water well and built-in tethering ports for deep-water exercises.

Guidelines for the Pool Program

Before you begin the pool program in Chapter 7, give some consideration to the physical limitations imposed by your hip. You'll want to be mindful of its condition each time you're in the pool and adjust your session accordingly.

- ***Let your body tell you which exercises you can do.*** Your body's pain messages are the best guide you have while exercising. Listen carefully. Don't expect your body to tell you the same thing every day, for the location and severity of your pain can change.

- *If you feel a sharp pain, stop what you're doing immediately.* Try making the same movement at a much slower pace. If that doesn't eliminate the pain, narrow the range of motion of that exercise. If moving more slowly or working through a narrower range of motion doesn't bring your pain level down significantly, *don't do that particular exercise yet.* Try it again slowly next week.
- *Respect the weakest link in your body "chain."* Your hip is the weak link at the moment. Any exercise program should move at the pace tolerated by that hip.
- *Underdo anything new.* Begin slowly, monitoring carefully for possible pain. Because you feel less pain in the water, and because you may not feel the pain of a new movement until the next day, perform fewer repetitions than you think you can tolerate and at a slower pace.
- *Perform all of your pool hip exercises gently, smoothly, and with correct biomechanics.* You may want to ask a therapist, a coach, or a knowledgeable friend to supervise you until you are sure all movements are exact. Follow the basic rules of good biomechanics listed below.
- *Do it first in the water!* Whatever you may be planning to do on land, try it out first in the pool, where you'll be less likely to harm your hip. Try a golf or tennis swing, try bending and reaching as you would at work. Remind your body what you expect of it before adding gravity.

Correct Biomechanics

Whether you sit, stand, walk, run, or perform any other activity, there is a position, posture, stance, or alignment that helps the body perform the activity most smoothly and with the least effort or strain. If you use correct biomechanics, good form, your movements will be more efficient. When you first begin your pool program, focus on good form before adding speed.

Here are some general rules of good biomechanics:

- *Never work faster than your form will allow.* If your form crumbles during any of the exercises, particularly the deep-water running and walking, slow down, and put the building blocks together again from the beginning.
- *Imagine a string attached to the top of your head and a helium balloon lifting it straight up toward the sky or ceiling.* This will help you walk and run tall. Keep your chest lifted and your shoulders relaxed and down.
- *Find a focal point at eye level.* By keeping your eyes focused on that point, your head will be less likely to bob or weave. Holding your head steady helps you keep your shoulders and hips steady. If your chin tilts up, your back automatically arches and the hips sway back. If your chin tilts down, your body tends to curl inward.
- *Notice the position of your feet.* They should remain parallel, toes pointing forward throughout all the movements unless otherwise specified.
- *Try to isolate the muscles involved in each exercise.* Don't move other body parts to generate a "whipping" action for added strength. For example, when doing leg circles, many people swing their entire bodies in order to move the legs. Instead, hold the rest of your body stable while you use only the muscles surrounding the hip to do the work. That way you'll gain more strength exactly where you targeted it.

Improving Your Pool Workouts

Here are some tips for improving your pool workouts:

- Establish your space in the pool.
- Ignore curious onlookers.
- Keep your goals firmly in mind.
- Concentrate on your movements.
- Have fun in the water.

7

A Pool Program
for Hip Patients

You can gain at least one wonderful, perhaps unexpected, benefit from exercising your unhealthy hip. If you are willing to commit to the following aquatic therapy program, your entire body will eventually be in great shape. You will become stronger and more flexible, have better cardiovascular capacity, move more efficiently, and will simply feel better.

This program keeps in mind three categories of people:

- Those who are trying to prevent hip surgery
- Those who are recovering from hip arthroscopy (see Chapter 11)
- Those who are recovering from hip implant surgery (see Chapter 12)

The basic instructions are intended for everyone unless specific warnings or other instructions are included. *Those recovering from hip implant surgery should read the box at the end of the chapter.*

If you're comfortable in deep water, put on your flotation vest or belt and begin with Exercise 1. (See page 64 for guidance in selecting a flotation device.) Your program contains exercises in both deep and shallow water. If you're a nonswimmer or afraid of the water, move straight to Exercise 5. You'll start in shallow water and won't need a flotation belt. Over time you will gain confidence in the water and may be able to add Exercises 1 to 4 to your program.

Deep Exercises

Exercise 1. Deep-Water Running

Run in an upright position using the exact motion of good running form on land. Lift each knee, then push each foot straight down behind you, following the path of the arrow in Photo 23. Focus your eyes on a point straight ahead that will help you keep your head level and unmoving. Keep your chest erect and your shoulders relaxed and down. Lift each knee so that your thigh is at a 90-degree angle to your body, or as high as your hip will allow if 90 degrees causes you pain. Pull your arms forward and backward with no lateral movement. Relax your hands, palms facing inward, not down, and pull your elbows straight back, each in its turn. Don't lean too far forward or you'll be dog-paddling. Don't lean too far back or you'll start kicking into a bicycling motion (Photo 24).

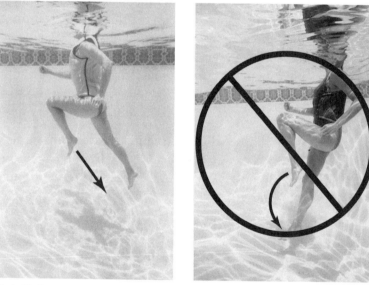

Photo 23. Deep-water running (Wet Vest shown).

Photo 24. Deep-water running, too far back (Wet Vest II shown).

Recovering from hip implant surgery: If you feel tentative about moving your hip in this way, start your warm-up holding on to the pool for stability (Photo 25). Or you can use hand buoys or a therapy bar to give you a greater sense of security, as shown in Photo 26.

Don't lift your knees as high as the 90 degrees shown in Photo 23. Start gradually, barely lifting your knees and stopping at the level at which you feel comfortable. Don't let your knees turn in, crossing the midline of the body.

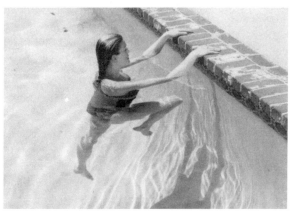

Photo 25. Holding the side of the pool to begin deep-water running (Wet Belt shown).

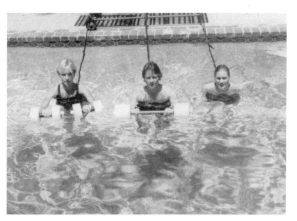

Photo 26. Using Waterpower Workout tethers to stay in place and Hydro-Fit Hand Buoys and Therapy Bar if needed for balance.

Start Deep-Water Walking Slowly

Begin Exercise 2, Deep-Water Walking, slowly. A lot of force is required to swing straight legs through the water's resistance. It is possible to strain your hip flexor muscles from working too fast too soon, so increase your speed very gradually over several weeks.

Exercise 2. Deep-Water Walking—Power Walk, Speed Walk

Start in an upright position with no forward or backward lean. Hold your right arm and your left leg forward at the same time to establish your "opposition" position (Photo 27). Then begin an exaggerated walking motion, one in which the knees *never* bend. Swing your arms and legs forward and backward—right arm with left leg and left arm with right leg—in a smooth, flowing motion.

Power walk. Turn your hands so the palms face backward and they're wide like paddles. This creates increased resistance for your shoulders, chest, and back. In order to create more work for your calf muscles, flex the foot on the leg that swings forward and point the foot on the leg that swings backward. One foot is flexing and one is pointing on each step (Photo 28).

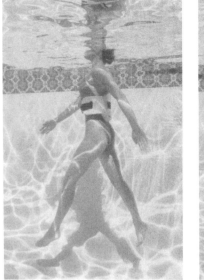

Photo 27. Deep-water walking (AquaJogger shown).

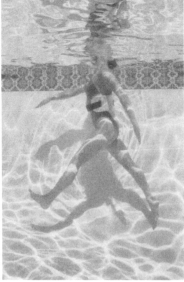

Photo 28. Power walk (AquaJogger shown).

Speed walk. Turn your hands with the thumbs forward so that they "slice" through the water. Your elbows and knees remain straight throughout the exercise. Tighten your abdominal muscles and your gluteal (buttocks) muscles to create a solid torso from which to rapidly swing your arms and legs. Lift your toes so that your feet are flat as if you were standing on land. (This will help you keep your knees straight.) Narrow the forward and backward range of motion of your legs so they swing forward and backward less than a foot or so (Photo 29). Now quicken your steps as you carefully hold your op-position position. If your shoulders begin to wobble, you've lost the opposition. Slow down and start again, gradually building the speed.

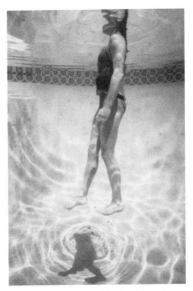

Photo 29. Speed walk (Wet belt shown).

Recovering from hip implant surgery: Stick with the basic walking maneuver for the first two to three weeks. Very gradually introduce Power Walk into your program, but if you feel undue strain in the hip flexors, quads, or hamstrings, return to the basic walk and try again in two weeks. Wait until six weeks after your surgery before trying Speed Walk. If the quick movements cause you deep hip pain joint, slow down. Over the next weeks and months you can increase the speed.

Exercise 3. Flies

Assume the "T" position shown in Photo 30 with your hands to the sides and your feet together. Now pull your arms together and swing your legs to the open position shown in Photo 31. Return with equal force to the starting position.

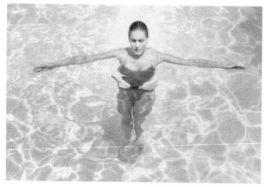

Photo 30. Flies, T position (Speedo belt shown).

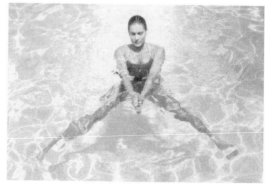

Photo 31. Flies, open position.

Recovering from hip implant surgery: Some orthopedic surgeons allow their patients to perform abduction and adduction (opening and closing) of the hips within two weeks of surgery. Others ask you to refrain from this movement for up to twelve weeks. Different surgical techniques and implants require different postsurgical practices, so ask your doctor when you can begin this exercise.

Deep-Water Interval Training

You will use the skills you learned in Exercises 1 through 3 to create a powerful cardiovascular series. At the same time you'll be developing good biomechanics while you strengthen all the muscles that surround your hips.

Interval training involves performing a challenging work period, then resting, then working again. Running and Walking are used as the work periods, while Flies are used as the recovery periods. At first you may not be challenging your cardiovascular system and may not require much of a rest period. However, as your hip heals and can withstand more force, you'll be able to increase the effort and speed of these intervals and raise your working heart rate to whatever level you desire.

All of these intervals start with low intensity and move to higher intensity. *If you feel an increase in pain in your hip at any time, slow down.* If you have any concerns for your heart, discuss this program with your physician before beginning and monitor your heart rate where suggested.

Measuring Your Heart Rate

To measure your heart rate, count the number of beats you feel at your carotid artery in your neck for six seconds. Add a zero to find your heart rate. Not only is this the easiest way to compute your heart rate, but recent studies have shown it to be more accurate than counting for ten seconds and multiplying by six.

Exercise 4. Interval Training

Preventing hip surgery: Do the medium-intensity program the first session. If it seems too difficult, move back to low intensity right away. If it seems too easy, don't move up to the high-intensity program until the next session. You won't know until the next day whether your hip or your muscles are going to be sore or whether you will become overly fatigued.

Recovering from hip arthroscopy: Do the low-intensity program the first two weeks, then progress to the medium-intensity program during weeks three and four. If you feel undue pain in your hip from increasing the speed of movement, return to the low-intensity program for another two weeks before trying to progress again. Use that same rule of thumb in another month or two if you wish to progress to the high-intensity program.

Recovering from hip implant surgery: Do the low-intensity program for the first six to eight weeks. When this program starts to feel too easy, try the medium-intensity program. If you feel undue pain in your hip from increasing the speed of movement, return to the low-intensity program for another two weeks before trying to progress again. Use that same rule of thumb in another few months if you wish to progress to the high-intensity program.

Low-Intensity Program
>   Water run (slow), one minute
>   Basic walk or power walk (slow), one minute
>   Flies (Exercise 3), thirty seconds
>   Water run (slow), two minutes
>   Basic walk or power walk (slow), two minutes
>   (Heart-rate check)
>   Flies, thirty seconds

Repeat this sequence once or twice per your tolerance.
Total time: 7 minutes, once, 14 minutes (if repeated), or 21 minutes (if repeated twice)

Medium-Intensity Program
>   Water run (slow), one minute
>   Water run (moderate), one minute
>   Flies, thirty seconds
>   Water run (slow), one minute

Water run (moderate), one minute
Basic Walk or power walk (moderate), one minute
(Heart-rate check)
Flies, thirty seconds
Basic walk or power walk (slow), one minute
Basic walk or power walk (moderate), one minute
Water run (moderate), one minute
(Heart-rate check)
Flies, thirty seconds
Power walk (slow), thirty seconds
Speed walk (fast), thirty seconds
Flies, thirty seconds
(Heart-rate check)

Repeat this sequence if your stamina and your hip allow.
Total time: 11 minutes or 22 minutes (if repeated)

High-Intensity Program

Even if your fitness level can handle a high-intensity series of intervals, you must re-member to defer to your hip. If working fast and hard against the water resistance in-creases the pain in your hip, *slow down.* If running is easier on your hip than walking, do your fastest, hardest intervals in running mode and your slower and more moderate intervals while walking. Skip speed walk altogether if it causes too much pain. Over the weeks, try gradually to introduce speed walk to your program.

Water run, one-minute buildup, increasing pace every fifteen seconds to create a
    four-speed interval: slow, medium, fast, sprint.
(Heart-rate check)
Flies, thirty seconds
Repeat one-minute buildup: slow, medium, fast, sprint
(Heart-rate check)
Flies, thirty seconds
Power walk (moderate), one minute
Power walk (hard), thirty seconds
(Heart-rate check)
Flies, thirty seconds
Power walk (moderate), one minute
Speed walk (fast), thirty seconds

(Heart-rate check)
Flies, thirty seconds
Run (fast), thirty seconds
Power walk (hard), thirty seconds
Speed walk (fast), thirty seconds
(Heart-rate check)
Flies, thirty seconds
Run (fast), one minute
Power walk (hard), one minute
Speed walk (fast), thirty seconds
(Heart-rate check)
Flies, thirty seconds

Repeat this sequence if your stamina and your hip allow.
Total time: twelve minutes or twenty-four minutes (if repeated)

Gradually increase the difficulty of your interval session over the next weeks and months. Use what you've learned about interval training from the examples above to create your own personalized interval session that lasts fifteen to thirty minutes. Vary your session from day to day to avoid losing interest.

Shallow or Deep

Kick Training

Exercises 5 to 8 offer you a variety of exercises that target the hips, thighs, and buttocks for strengthening. You can do them in deep water or in shallow water, with or without a flotation belt. If you skipped Exercises 1 to 4 because you didn't want to work in deep water, begin here in shallow water without a flotation belt. If you've already done Exercises 1 to 4, the most logical progression is to keep your flotation belt on and stay in deep water for Exercises 5 to 8 in this section.

Find the most comfortable position for your arms on the gutter or lip of the pool. That position may change from exercise to exercise. Experiment to keep your shoulders comfortable. You may prefer to do all these kicks on the steps of your pool.

Exercise 5. Deep Back Kicks

Grasp the side of the pool, the gutter, or a ladder. Lean forward and look down at the water. Let your hips float near the surface of the water and let your left leg dangle below you (Photo 32). Lift your right leg straight back, but not so high as to arch your back. Now switch leg positions and keep reswitching smoothly, taking care to hold your hips steady. Don't let them roll from side to side. Focus on moving *only* your straight legs. Each right-left sequence counts as one repetition. Do ten to twenty reps.

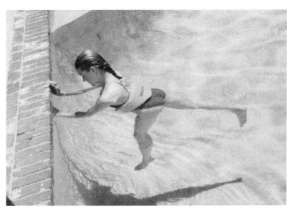

Photo 32. Deep back kicks (Speedo belt shown).

Recovering from hip implant surgery: Start with a narrow range of motion at first by minimizing the backward push; be absolutely certain your feet don't break the surface of the water. Even though most of your postsurgical warnings restrict you from too much flexion (forward bending), you must also avoid extreme extension (backward reaching) movements for the first six to eight weeks.

Exercise 6. Flutter Kick—Back/Front

Brace yourself with your back to the pool wall and your arms on the gutter or edge of the pool. Lift your hips and legs and begin shallow flutter kicks with straight legs. If you do your kicking series on a step or ledge, stay low in the water, as shown in Photo 33. Do thirty to forty right-left repetitions.

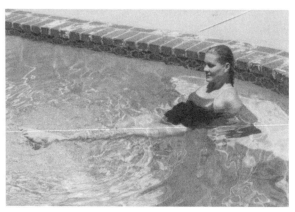

Photo 33. Back flutter kicks (H.A.N. model Wet Belt shown).

Now turn over and brace yourself facing the side of the pool with your legs floating behind you toward the surface of the water. Hold the pool lip or gutter with one hand and place the other hand a foot lower to provide maximum leverage for keeping your legs afloat. Begin tiny flutter kicks with straight legs. If you do your flutter kicks on a step or ledge, bend your elbows so your shoulders are under the water and you don't strain your back. Do thirty to forty left-right repetitions.

Recovering from hip implant surgery: Don't force your feet to break the surface of the water during front or back flutter kicking. Your legs will probably feel more comfortable working below the water.

Exercise 7. Bicycling

Brace yourself at the side of the pool and bend your knees to begin kicking in a bicycling movement (see Photo 1, page 3). Do twenty to thirty right-left repetitions.

Recovering from hip implant surgery: Don't lift your knees above 90 degrees. In fact, your knees may not even break the surface of the water. Over the months, your knee lift will naturally increase. Don't force it.

Exercise 8. Hip Openers

If you're wearing a belt, let your body continue to float slightly away from the pool wall. If you're not wearing a belt, push your lower back against the side of the pool and brace yourself as shown in Photo 2 on page 3. Open your legs wide (Photo 3, page 3), then close them again. Continue opening and closing them, using as much force in opening the legs as you use in closing them.

Recovering from hip arthroscopy: During the first two weeks after surgery, perform this exercise slowly. During weeks three and four, gradually apply more force as you push against the water. If you have no undue pain, you can continue gradually increasing the speed and power of the exercise.

Recovering from hip implant surgery: Ask your doctor or therapist when you can begin this exercise. Over the weeks you will find your legs naturally floating to a wider and wider position, so don't feel you have to force them. Your range of motion will automatically increase as nature heals your hip.

Shallow Program

Those who have been in deep water should now move to the shallow end of the pool for the rest of the program.

Gait Training

You may have damaged your hip in a sudden injury, or it may have taken months or years for your hip condition to develop. Either way, you have probably found that your normal walking pattern has become irregular due to pain or limitation of the hip's movement. If walking on land causes you hip pain or discomfort, you'll find it a welcome relief to have most of your weight lifted off your hip joint while you walk in the water. In chest-deep water, you can walk relatively pain-free and at the same time relearn or refine the correct biomechanics of walking. (See page 72 for more on biomechanics.)

If your pool bottom is slippery or if your feet tend to blister easily, wear Speedo Surfwalkers or other pool shoes to provide traction and protection. If you have diabetes, rheumatoid arthritis, or have had a hip implant operation, *always* wear pool shoes to prevent a cut that could become infected.

Walk back and forth across the width of a pool if possible, so that you will have the same depth of water and same amount of water resistance throughout the exercise. You can still get the job done if you must walk the length of the pool in one lane, but you will find yourself constantly adjusting to a changing amount of buoyancy and resistance due to the changing depth of the water. (See page 68 for an explanation of the importance of finding a pool with an unslanted bottom that has the correct depth of water for gait training.)

Before performing Exercises 9 to 12, spend a moment trying to visualize yourself walking tall, straight, and without any limp or deviation in your gait. Picture your feet and knees always facing forward and your hips and shoulders always level, never rocking up and down or from side to side. Then begin with Exercise 9. Perform each of the walking exercises for one or two pool crossings during the first few sessions. Increase over the next weeks.

Recovering from hip arthroscopy: Hip pain may have altered your normal walking pattern prior to surgery. Although the presurgical pain may have been eliminated, you could be surprised to find that you are still limping. If this is the case, your limp is just a bad habit that it's time to break. Your normal walking pattern will have to be rebuilt with these exercises. Spend extra time on gait training until an observer—a partner, coach, or aquatic therapist—says you are walking normally again.

Recovering from hip implant surgery: Make sure the pool you use as you begin these exercises will have a relatively unslanted bottom. If the pool is steeply slanted, you'll find yourself walking with one leg functionally longer than the other. You don't want that, so drive the extra few miles to a pool that will provide you with a level pool bottom.

Wear a flotation belt or vest as you take your first walking steps in chest-deep water. Keep the belt on until you feel confident of your walking skills and are no longer limping *at all.* Your normal walking pattern will have to be rebuilt with these exercises. Spend extra time on gait training until an observer—a partner, coach, or aquatic therapist—says you are walking normally again. When walking across the pool, *start your turn at the side by leading with the postsurgical leg.* In that way you won't inadvertently turn your leg into internal rotation. (See Photo 68, page 163.)

Modifications If You Feel Pain

If you feel pain in the unhealthy hip when you step on it, try these basic modifications:

1. Move to slightly deeper water.
2. Take smaller steps.
3. Strap on your flotation belt.

Exercise 9. Shallow Water Walking—Backward, Forward, Sideways

Walking *backward* in water is easier than walking forward, so you will start by walking backward. Face the side of the pool and prepare to take your first small steps onto the sore or postsurgical hip. Look to see that you have an unobstructed space behind you, then begin walking backward. Don't worry about your arms while walking backward. If you feel pain when you step on the unhealthy hip, try the basic modifications shown in the box above. Walk slowly across the pool, turn, and continue walking backward across the pool again. Keep your steps short until you can walk without a limp, then gradually lengthen them. After crossing the pool several times, try walking forward.

Face the center of the pool and prepare to walk *forward,* taking a small step onto your leg with the sore hip. Hold the opposite arm forward to establish an opposition position. Take first one small step, then another, moving your arms and legs in time with each other. Once again, if you feel pain in the unhealthy hip when you step on it, try the basic modifications. Make sure your right arm moves with your left leg and your left arm moves with your right leg. If this cross-crawl patterning (see page 63) is too difficult to master right now, let your arms float comfortably at your sides for balance. Eventually you do want to learn to walk with opposition between your arms and legs, but that isn't your first priority—walking without a limp is. Cross the pool several times walking with small steps until all gait irregularities are gone. Then you can begin lengthening your steps.

Next walk *sideways* across the pool, starting by pushing off with your healthiest side and stepping onto the sore side. Bring the healthy leg to a closed position. Step and close, step and close in this manner across the pool, starting with small steps. Look down at your feet. Many people incorrectly turn their feet in the direction they are stepping. *Constantly check your feet to make sure they are parallel and pointing straight forward.* If you encounter any pain, move to deeper water, take smaller steps, or put on your flotation belt. Don't lurch or lean from side to side. Rather, keep your shoulders and hips level throughout the sideways walking. When you've crossed the pool, *keep facing in the same direction,* so that as you recross the pool, you will this time push off with the opposite leg.

A Helpful Visualization

Some patients have had bad gait patterns for so many years that they feel quite normal lurching from side to side as they walk. Even in chest-deep water they limp badly, and can't quite conceptualize what a normal gait would be. Try this visualization: Pretend that the sides of your body are made of steel and that a bell hangs straight down the center of your body on a string attached to your head. If you lean to the right, the bell will clang noisily against the right steel wall, and if you lean to the left, it will clang against the left steel wall. Do everything in your power to keep that bell hanging straight down from your head, not swinging from side to side.

Exercise 10. Marching

Begin marching by lifting a knee to the position shown in Photo 34, or as high as you can before you feel undue hip pain. Lean forward and take a step, then lift the other knee up to a similar position. If you feel pain in the unhealthy hip and you've tried the basic modifications in the box on page 89, don't lift your knee so high. Pay attention to the direction your knees are pointing while you march. Perhaps your right knee is pointing straight forward while your left knee points slightly to the left side or across the midline of your body. Try to correct the movement so that *both knees point straight forward.* If the correction causes increased hip pain, make a note to tell your doctor. Continue *aiming* toward correct biomechanics but only to the point at which you feel a slight discomfort, no real pain. Use bent arms in opposition to the bent knees. Your right arm should move in time with your left knee, and your left arm should move with your right knee.

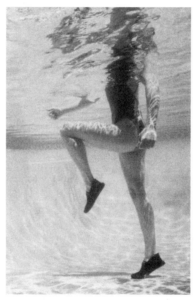

Photo 34. Marching, knee to ninety degrees.

Recovering from hip implant surgery: Lift your knee to only 45 degrees—half as high as the 90 degrees shown in Photo 34. Over the weeks and months your knee will begin to rise up toward 90 degrees by itself. Don't force it. Do *not* let your knee cross the midline of the body.

Exercise 11. Long-Leg Walk

Walking forward, lift your straight right leg toward the surface of the water and reach your left arm forward for balance and opposition (Photo 35). Continue this long-leg walk across the pool, swinging your arms forcefully through the water in opposition to your legs.

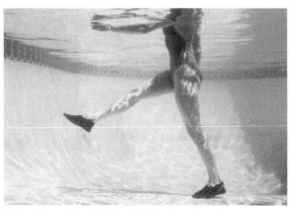

Photo 35. Long-leg walk (Speedo Surfwalkers shown).

Recovering from hip implant surgery: Skip this exercise until all the other gait-training exercises have become easy and you are walking without a limp. When you add it, move slowly and lift each leg only as high as you comfortably can. Over time the leg will start lifting higher without your having to force it.

Exercise 12. Bouncing—Backward, Forward

Bouncing backward is easier than bouncing forward, so start backward. Face the side of the pool, slowly bend both knees, and lower yourself to a half-squat position. Gently straighten both legs at the same time and take a small jump backward. Immediately bend both knees again and smoothly continue bouncing backward across the pool. Now try bouncing forward.

When you feel ready, try bouncing backward then forward on just one leg. Try the healthier leg first, then gently try the recovering one. If you feel undue pain, simply lift your leg and let the water catch you. You might not be ready for one-legged bounces yet. Try again in another week or two.

Recovering from hip implant surgery: Skip this exercise until all the others have become easy and you are walking without a limp. When you add it, wear a flotation belt when you first attempt bouncing backward. If you aren't comfortable with the thought of trying this one, *don't.*

Stretching

Stretching reduces muscle tension and makes your body feel more relaxed. It increases the range of motion of your hip joint while it helps you get to know your own body better: as you stretch, you receive messages from your body. Listen to these messages carefully.

Never force a stretch if there is pain. Stretch only to the point of discomfort to find your limit. Then ease back a bit and hold a challenging stretching position while you breathe slowly and deeply to assist the stretching process.

Turn to face the side of the pool for stretching exercises 13 to 16. If you perform them in deep water, wear a flotation device. If you do them in shallow water, you won't need one.

Is One Side More Flexible?

Don't be surprised to find that one leg or one side of your body is more flexible than the other. You can address that imbalance by spending more time stretching the tight side. The easiest way to do that is to stretch the tight side first, then the other side, then return to the tight side for a final stretch.

Exercise 13. Hamstring Stretch

Grasp the side of the pool, a gutter, or a ladder with both hands, or if you have an Aqua-Trend Pool Bar, insert it through your skimmer box as shown in Photo 36. Place your left foot, toes up, against the pool wall. Keep your neck, shoulders, arms, and back relaxed throughout the exercise. Gently straighten your left knee as far as you can while you breathe deeply and slowly five times. Over the next weeks and months try to push your left heel to make contact with the pool wall.

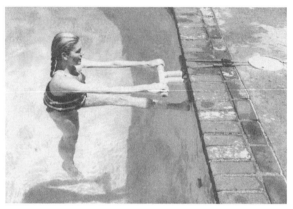

Photo 36. Hamstring stretch (AquaTrend Pool Bar and Hydro-Tone belt shown).

Recovering from hip implant surgery: Lift your leg to only 45 degrees (at least one foot lower on the wall than in Photo 36), and bend your knee slightly if you must. Do not lean your head or chest forward. Maintain a focal point straight in front of you so that your head and chest will be upright.

Exercise 14. Lateral Split

Continue grasping the side of the pool or an AquaTrend Pool Bar. Gradually walk your feet away from each other, opening your legs to the side as far as you comfortably can (see Photo 9 on page 6). If the position is too comfortable, stretch slightly further. If the position is painfully uncomfortable, move your feet closer together. Hold this position while you take five slow deep breaths. As you improve at this stretch, you can make it more difficult by leaning your upper body forward toward the pool wall.

Recovering from hip implant surgery: Some surgeons ask you not to do any hip abduction (opening of the legs) during the first few months after surgery. In that case, skip this exercise until the appropriate time. When you add it, drop your feet at least a foot down the wall before very gently opening your legs comfortably apart. Do *not* force this stretch, and do not lean forward for at least six to eight weeks.

Exercise 15. Quad Stretch

Hold the side of the pool for balance with your right hand. Grasp your left ankle with your left hand and slowly pull the left heel toward the buttocks as shown in Photo 37. Keep the knees close together and make sure you haven't gone into a swayback position. Breathe deeply five times as you feel the muscles relax and lengthen. Switch sides. Hold onto the side of the pool with your left hand and repeat with the right leg.

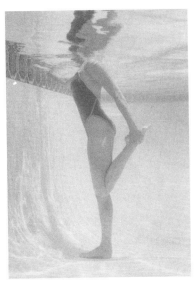

Recovering from hip implant surgery: You may not be able to assume this position for several months after surgery. Once you can reach the position in Photo 37, hold it right there. Don't let your knee drift backward toward the position shown in Photo 38 until you get your surgeon's permission.

Photo 37. Quad stretch.

Exercise 16. Hip Flexor Stretch

If you have a lower-back problem, ask your doctor or therapist if you can do this exercise.

Start in the same position as for Exercise 15. *Keep your left elbow straight* as you allow your left knee to swing straight backward to the position shown in Photo 38. Look up at the ceiling to further increase the stretch of the hip flexors. Breathe slowly and deeply five times, then repeat on the other side.

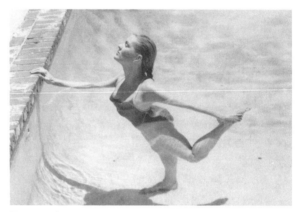

Photo 38. Hip flexor stretch.

Recovering from hip arthroscopy: Try this stretch gently at first. If you have undue pain, wait two weeks before trying again.

Recovering from hip implant surgery: Skip this exercise for at least eight weeks. Before adding this exercise, get permission from your doctor or therapist. When you do, move slowly and carefully and release the position immediately if you feel any undue pain or discomfort.

Waterpower Workout Exercises

As you gain strength and flexibility in your hip, you might be tempted to return to your normal land activities. Before you do, try these gentle impact exercises to see if your hip is ready for an even greater weight-bearing load on land. If you experience hip pain during or after these exercises, you aren't yet ready to return to land. Continue to prepare your hip for land activities by increasing the number of repetitions you do of each exercise and by increasing the intensity of your running. (See "Lynda Huey's Waterpower Workout" video or *The Complete Waterpower Workout Book* by Lynda Huey and Robert Forster, P.T., for a complete series of shallow-water exercises.)

Recovering from hip arthroscopy: Wait until you've had no weight-bearing pain in your hip for at least two weeks before attempting to add these exercises to your program. If they cause you any discomfort, put on a flotation belt and try again.

Recovering from hip implant surgery: Don't begin the Waterpower Workout Exercise until you've mastered everything else in the program without increasing your hip pain. These are jumping and running exercises and should be introduced only at the end of your rehab program. Wear your flotation device the first few times to gain confidence in your ability to withstand the impact.

Exercise 17. Lunges

Assume the lunge position shown in Photo 39 with your right knee forward and bent. Your left leg is straight and to the rear. Your left arm is forward for counterbalance. Jump up and switch arm and leg positions so that the left leg is now forward and the right arm is forward. Make sure your right arm is forward with your left leg and your left arm is forward with your right leg. Each right-left cycle is one repetition. Start with only ten reps the first time, then if your hip remains pain-free, add two reps each week until you've reached twenty reps. Once you've reached twenty reps, start jumping higher, increasing the impact placed on your hip.

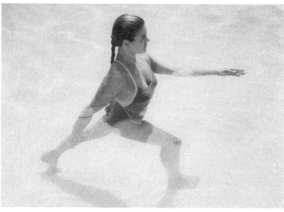

Photo 39. Lunges.

Exercise 18. Power Frog Jumps

Bounce gently with your feet together and your arms out to your sides at chest level. Jump off both feet and lift both knees toward your chest as you sweep both arms forward

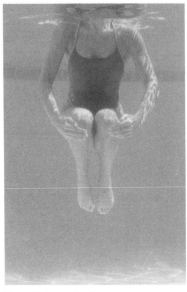

to meet in front of you (Photo 40). Push the arms back to their starting position as your feet return to the pool bottom. Start with ten and work to twenty reps, then start jumping higher.

Recovering from hip implant surgery: Don't lift your knees as high as shown in Photo 40. Lift them only as high as you feel you can with confidence. Over time your knees will naturally start lifting higher as your hip heals.

Photo 40. Power frog jumps.

Exercise 19. Running

Begin running in place, simulating good running form on land. (Do not run across the pool, because that creates entirely different forces on your body and hip.) The head and chest are erect and the eyes look straight ahead. The shoulders stay down and stable without rocking side to side. Lift your knees and pull your arms directly forward and back without any lateral movement. Make sure you are using opposition: your right arm is forward with your left knee and your left arm is forward with your right knee.

Once you've established good running form, begin increasing your speed. If your form breaks down, slow down and correct your biomechanics. Then pick up the pace again. When your hip has been pain-free at least two weeks, try these sample intervals. A work period is followed by a slower recovery period, then another work period until you've completed two to five minutes of running. Monitor your heart rate where noted.

Preventing hip surgery: Do the medium-intensity intervals the first session. If they seem too difficult, move back to low intensity right away. If they seem too easy, don't move up to high intensity until the next session. You won't know until tomorrow if your muscles or hip are going to be sore or if you will become overly fatigued.

Recovering from hip arthroscopy: Don't add shallow-water running to your program until you've had at least two weeks without hip pain. Begin with the medium-intensity intervals.

Recovering from hip implant surgery: Running in chest-deep water can be added near the end of your rehab program. Once you begin, do the low-intensity intervals for the first two weeks. When this program starts to feel too easy for both you and your hip, try the medium-intensity intervals. If you feel undue pain in your hip from increasing the speed of movement, return to low intensity for another two weeks before trying to progress again. Use that same rule of thumb in another month or two if you wish to progress to the high-intensity intervals.

Low-Intensity Program

    Run (easy), one to two minutes
    Walk across the pool and back
    Run (easy), one to two minutes
    (Heart-rate check)

Medium-Intensity Program

    Run (easy), one minute
    Run (medium or fast), thirty seconds
    Run (easy), thirty seconds
    Run (medium or fast), forty-five seconds
    Run (easy), thirty seconds
    Run (medium), one minute
    (Heart-rate check)

Repeat this sequence if you wish.

High-Intensity Program

    Tether yourself to a railing or a ladder on the side of the pool when running at high speeds. This allows you to remain stable and focus on your workload instead of constantly adjusting your position. (See page 67 for more about the Waterpower Workout Tether.) If you can't find anything to tether to, you can tie a rope to a nearby tree or ask a training partner to hold the end.

    Run (easy), thirty seconds
    Run (sprint), thirty seconds
    (Heart-rate check)

Repeat the above sequence two more times.

    Run (easy), thirty seconds
    Run (sprint), forty-five seconds
    (Heart-rate check)

Repeat this sequence two more times.

Gradually increase the difficulty of your interval session over the next weeks and months. If you are preparing to return to golf, tennis, or other land activities, you can eliminate the deep-water intervals and focus your time and effort on the shallow-water intervals. Use what you've learned about interval training from the examples above to create your own personalized interval session that lasts ten to twenty minutes. Vary it from day to day to avoid losing interest.

> If I could tell you only one thing about mainintaining hip function, it would be this: *Demand as much motion from your hip joint as possible.*
> —*Robert Klapper, M.D.*

Lower Extremity Exercises

If you feel any pain during these exercises, *slow down or narrow the range of motion.* You'll start your program using only the water's resistance against your legs. As your strength improves, you can add one of three pieces as your individual needs dictate. Try a Hydra-Flow Water Weight (see page 66) if you need moderate buoyancy and resistance. Move slowly as you feel it lift your leg higher than usual, but also require more muscular effort as you move your leg. When you become familiar with that feeling, progress to a Hydro-Fit Cuff (see page 67) for maximum buoyancy and maximum assistance with range of motion. Finally, use a Hydro-Tone boot (see page 66) for maximum resistance to increase your strength. (All three pieces are shown in Photo 42 on page 101.)

Keep in mind that your hip can feel different every day, so you must adjust your workload accordingly. *If your hip is painful, don't use the resistance equipment.* Save the extra resistance for days when your hip and the muscles around it are feeling pain-free and eager for more work.

Notice if your sore hip is not capable of as much motion as your healthier hip. In that case, you may decide to do more repetitions on the sore side to try to bring it slowly back to full function. The easiest way to do more work on one side is to do all your exercises on the sore leg, do a second set on the healthy side, then go back to the sore side for a third set.

Recovering from hip implant surgery: You may not be able to stand on your post-surgical leg to do these exercises for several weeks. In that case, work only the postsurgical leg while standing on the healthy leg. Do the exercises on both legs as soon as possible.

Exercise 20. Lateral Leg Raises

Stand with your right hand on the side of the pool facing the end of the pool (Photo 41). Maintain erect posture and lift your left leg directly to the side (Photo 42). Don't lean to the side to be able to lift your leg higher. Keep the feet parallel so that your left knee points forward rather than upward. Pull your left leg back to the starting position. Apply equal force as you lift the leg up and pull it down. Do ten to twenty reps, then turn and repeat with the right leg. When twenty reps becomes easy, try adding a Hydra-Flow Water Weight, a Hydro-Fit Cuff, or a Hydro-Tone Boot.

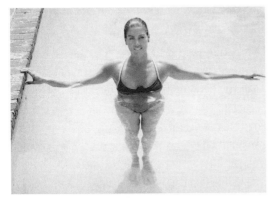

Photo 41. Lateral leg raises, starting position.

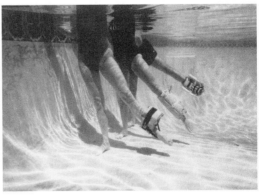

Photo 42. Lateral leg raises, leg lifted with (left to right) Hydro-Fit Cuff, Hydra-Flow Water Weight, Hydro-Tone Boot.

Recovering from hip implant surgery: Ask your doctor or therapist when you can begin this exercise. When you first begin it, don't lift your leg very high to the side, and *don't use any equipment.* Over the next weeks and months you'll find your leg naturally lifting higher and higher almost by itself.

Exercise 21. Leg Swings

To protect your lower back, tighten your abdominal and gluteal muscles as you do this exercise. Continue standing erect with your hand on the side of the pool for stability. Swing your left leg straight forward (see Photo 4, page 4), then swing it down and to the rear (see Photo 5, page 4). *If a full swing backward hurts your back, don't reach so far.* Do ten to twenty reps, then turn and repeat with the right leg. Once twenty reps are easy for you, try adding a Hydra-Flow Water Weight, a Hydro-Fit Cuff, or a Hydro-Tone Boot for buoyancy or resistance as needed.

Recovering from hip implant surgery: Don't try to lift your postsurgical leg as high as shown in the photos. Lift it only as high as is comfortable at first, and limit your backswing as well. Over the next weeks and months it will naturally start lifting higher by itself. Don't force it. Eventually you'll find yourself using your full range of motion.

Exercise 22. Leg Circles

If you have lower-back pain, make much smaller circles than shown in the photos on the next page.

Lift your left leg straight forward in front of you just as you began your leg swings (Photo 43). This time, however, smoothly sweep your leg in a circular motion by swinging the leg out to your left side (Photo 44), then behind you (Photo 45). Complete the circle by brushing your left leg past your right leg, then beginning the next large circle. Carefully monitor for pain that would tell you either to slow down or make your circles smaller. If you have no such pain, reach as far as you can in each direction. This is one of your most important exercises in attempting to regain full range of motion of your hip, for only in water can you perform this full circumduction of the hip against a smooth three-dimensional resistance.

Start with five circles in this counterclockwise direction before doing the same number clockwise. Over the next weeks build up gradually to doing twenty reps in each direction. Add a Hydra-Flow Water Weight, a Hydro-Fit Cuff, or a Hydro-Tone Boot to gain maximum range of motion and strength in this important exercise.

Recovering from hip arthroscopy: For the first few weeks your hip could be sore. In that case, limit the range of motion. Don't lift your leg as high as shown in the photos. Over the next month your leg will gradually start floating up toward 90 degrees on its own. When the pain has been gone a few weeks, try adding a Hydra-Flow Cuff or a Hydro-Tone Cuff to gain range of motion. When you have full range, add the Hydro-Tone Boot for maximum resistance.

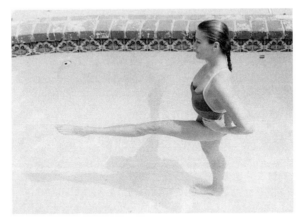

Photo 43. Leg circles, forward.

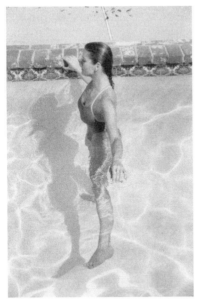

Photo 44. Leg circles, to side.

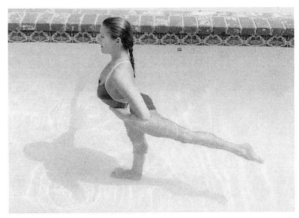

Photo 45. Leg circles, backward.

Recovering from hip implant surgery: Start leg circles only when your surgeon has allowed you to begin abduction and adduction. Although this exercise is actually circumduction (a circular motion), it combines elements of abduction and adduction. When you begin this exercise, don't lift your leg as high as shown in the photos. Make your circles with your foot along the pool bottom at first, then over the next weeks gradually lift your leg toward 45 degrees. It may be several months (or possibly never) before your hip lets your leg float up to the 90-degree position in the photos. Never force it; let the water do its magic by floating your leg higher and higher naturally.

Exercise 23. Internal and External Hip Rotations

Stand with your left knee bent and your thigh parallel to the surface of the water. For stability, tighten the muscles of your right leg and buttock. Turn your knee to the left into external rotation (see Photo 6, page 5), then to the right into internal rotation (see Photo 7, page 5). Do ten to twenty reps on each side, reaching as far as you can in each direction.

Recovering from implant surgery: Skip this exercise until your surgeon advises you that you no longer need to follow your hip precautions.

Exercise 24. Squats

Face the side of the pool in chest-deep water with your feet parallel and shoulder-width apart. Both hands grasp a gutter, ladder, or the lip of the pool. Focus your eyes on a point directly in front of you and maintain that focal point throughout the exercise. Keep your back straight and slowly bend both knees until you've lowered your chin to the water (see Photo 8 on page 5). Your heels may lift off the bottom at this point. Push your heels down as you stand up to the starting position. Start with ten reps, then work up to twenty to thirty reps.

Recovering from hip implant surgery: Wear your flotation belt as you perform this exercise. Lower yourself only as far as you feel comfortable on any given day. When you can easily do twenty reps, remove your flotation belt.

Hip Implant Patients

Get your surgeon's approval before beginning any new exercise program. Check with your physical therapist if you have concerns or questions about specific exercises. Be sure to comply with the basic hip precautions listed below that apply to your pool sessions. A more complete list of precautions appears on page 163. Warnings accompany certain exercises. Follow them carefully. You have a program that is limited for specific movements, and those limitations must be highly respected.

Hip Precautions
- Do not let your knee or ankle cross the midline of your body.
- Avoid hip flexion more than 90 degrees.
- Don't combine hip flexion with internal rotation (see Photo 67, page 163).
- When you reach the side of the pool after walking across it, always turn *away* from your postsurgical side to keep from forcing that hip into internal rotation (see Photo 68, page 163).
- If you drop your soap in the shower after your therapy session, *do not bend to pick it up.*

8

The Transition
from Pool to Land

"In water my hip doesn't hurt and my exercises feel so easy. Why do I need a land program at all?"

This is the question most frequently asked by patients who have been using the pool program to rehabilitate their hips, and of course the answer is, because you live on land, and also because

- you may have chlorine-sensitive skin
- some days you're simply stuck at home
- in a pool your ears may be prone to infection
- the pool may be unreasonably far from your home

But your main reason for exercising on land is that your *activities of daily living* (ADLs) take place there, not in buoyancy but in gravity. Get used to it! Get used to the earth's pull, which makes your movements different—and harder.

Picture an astronaut on the moon as he jumps, skips, and runs lightly across the surface in his gravity-reduced environment. When he returns to earth, the movements he performed with such ease become harder. More muscle fibers must fire to do the same tasks. He has to retrain himself to walk, jump, and do other physical activities against earth's gravity. You'll feel the same change as you move from the pool to land, as if you'd landed back on earth after being on the moon. Your body will feel heavier, and for a while you'll have to work harder to do the basic skills that were so easy in the pool.

Different laws of physics apply on land. That means different bio-mechanical rules apply as well—different laws of body movement. For instance, you don't walk the same in the water as you do on land. When you first tried walking in chest-deep water, you probably wobbled at first, having to learn new balance points as you pushed against the water's resistance. You used water's buoyancy to stand tall and walk without bobbing or lurching. As you corrected your gait pattern in the gravity-reduced environment of the water, you strengthened those muscles that are specific to good walking.

With that improved strength you can make the transition to land. The transition will take time—weeks or even months, depending on the severity of your gait abnormality. When you first try to duplicate your efficient pool alignment on land, you may not be able to maintain an upright posture because your muscles aren't yet strong enough. Yet each time that you reinforce your proper posture in the pool, then try again on land, you get closer to regaining a normal walking pattern. *Going back and forth from pool to land, pool to land, allows you to learn from both environments.* The water carries most of your weight while you focus on good posture and alignment; at the same time the water's resistance forces strength into the muscles specifically used for walking. Then on land you use the strength, posture, and alignment you developed in the pool to work against gravity.

The same holds true for your other activities of daily living. You took your ADLs for granted before your hip started hurting. Now every curb, ramp, or set of stairs can seem like a major obstacle to negotiate. You can relearn these movements that have become difficult on land by entering the water to reduce or eliminate gravity (your body's weight). In that way your body becomes skilled and strong in the functions necessary for your daily life on land. The result is improved **functionability,** which is the ability to function well within your specific environment. For instance, if you live in a house with seven steps, you need to be able to negotiate those steps without difficulty. You should be able to get safely into bed, the shower, and the bathtub, and in and out of the car and the easy chair. Yet hip pain often limits your ability to perform these basic activities.

Your job is to restore functionability so you can do the things your personal environment requires of you. If you need to be able to perform a specific movement that wasn't offered to you in Chapter 7, create your own pool exercise to generate the skill and strength that will eventually allow you to transition that movement onto land. For example, if it's difficult for you to vacuum your rug, simulate the vacuuming movement in the pool. After many repetitions, you'll be able to do that movement on land.

How to Get In and Out of Your Car

When a sore hip doesn't allow you much movement, getting in and out of a car can seem like a major accomplishment. Here's how to make it easy and as pain-free as possible.

Getting In
- Open the door.
- Turn and sit down on the car seat.
- Lift both knees and swing them together into the car.

Getting Out
- Scoot to the edge of the seat as far as possible.
- Open the door.
- Turn your torso and swing both legs at once to the side.
- Lean your trunk forward.
- Place your hands on the car and the door so you can use your upper body strength to assist you in standing.

Exercise Is Vital

Twenty years ago, exercise wasn't considered as vital as it is today. Research shows that exercise prevents many diseases, promotes good health, and is a key ingredient in any rehabilitation program. Not only does exercise speed the healing process, but studies have shown that a lack of exercise during the early stages of rehabilitation can actually cause permanent disability.

More specific to your hip, it has been demonstrated that muscular strength around a damaged joint can take over some of the joint's function. Instead of asking your hips to do all the work of supporting your body against gravity, strong muscles—your quadriceps, gluteals, hamstrings, abductors, and others—can do much of that job. If muscles provide a solid support around a hip joint, they take pressure off the weight-bearing surfaces by creating more joint space deep inside the hip, thus reducing friction on the damaged surfaces, and thereby reducing pain and slowing the deterioration.

Finding Balance

Although symmetry is emphasized in both the pool and land programs, the human body is not actually symmetrical to begin with—you probably have one foot or one hand that is slightly larger than the other. Degenerative changes to the body don't happen symmetrically either. Yet your body works symmetrically and your instincts are **bilateral.** You use both feet, both knees, both elbows, and both hips, and if you fall, both hands reach out to break your fall. Therefore your goal is to keep both sides of your body working efficiently. Both hips must be equally strong and limber: you should exercise both hips—the painful one to its maximum tolerance and your healthy hip just enough to keep it strong while the weaker one catches up.

Think about the last time you rode your bicycle when it was in disrepair. Perhaps the chain was loose and the pedals hesitated at every rotation. Maybe your wheels wobbled because the spokes needed bal-

Which Is Your Dominant Leg?

We all know we're right- or left-handed, but most people don't realize they also have a dominant right or left leg. Professional basketball players, Olympic high jumpers, and other top athletes are well aware that they have a favorite takeoff leg for jumping, and each of us has a preferred leg for movement, whether we know it or not. If your hip problem is your dominant leg, you might find that even a small amount of joint damage can cause severe limitations in your daily function, whereas if the problem hip is your nondominant leg, you might be able to live with that problem for a long time.

ancing. If you ignored your bike long enough, it might even have made a grinding sound in the bottom bracket where your pedals and crank arm are attached. The bike couldn't operate properly with all those parts malfunctioning, but once you tightened the chain, balanced the spokes of the wheels, and lubricated the bearings in the bottom bracket, you created harmony, stability, and balance. You got a smoother ride.

Your body also needs to be well maintained if you want a smooth ride through your daily activities. Your muscles work in synchronized pairs that need to be balanced. When half of a muscle pair contracts, the opposing one relaxes. The muscle pairs of the hip are the flexors/extensors, abductors/adductors, and internal rotators/external rotators. (See Drawings 3 to 6 on page 12.) Muscle pairs around a healthy hip retain a specific ratio of strength to each other; around an unhealthy hip that balance is lost. Most commonly, one-half a muscle pair becomes tight and restrictive while the other half becomes weak and overstretched.

The typical hip patient has tight adductors and weak abductors, tight flexors and weak extensors, and tight internal rotators and weak external rotators. To correct such imbalances, you need to stretch the tight muscles and strengthen the weak ones. Start by stretching the tight muscles first to increase your range of motion; then strengthen the weak muscles through the newly established range. If the warm-up stretches, Exercises 1 to 6 in Chapter 9, are painful or difficult, you may decide to visit a physical therapist who can help reduce your tightness and pain by performing the stretches for you.

Manual Stretches and Resistance Exercises

Every muscle has sensors embedded in the tissues. These sensors, the **muscle spindle** and the **golgi tendon organ,** tell the muscles and tendons what to do—when to contract (shorten) or when to relax (lengthen). If a muscle is stretched quickly, the spindle in the belly of the muscle will tell that muscle to contract against the stretch to maintain its usual length; but if a muscle is stretched very slowly with steady, uninterrupted pressure, the spindle stops asking for a contraction and the golgi tendon organ deep in the tendon starts asking the tissues to relax and lengthen to protect against being torn. The stretching technique discussed below works with these two sensors to produce positive results.

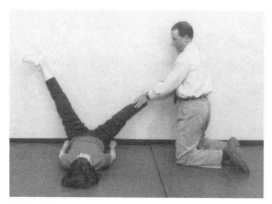

Photo 46. Passive, sustained stretch of right adductors by therapist.

If your right adductor muscles are tight, a physical therapist can apply a **passive, sustained stretch** by pulling your right leg to the side as far as it will reach and holding it there (Photo 46). You'll feel pain that will subside as the stretch is maintained for one to two minutes. As your muscles release, the therapist applies more pressure (within your pain tolerance) to constantly challenge the hip to its new, increased range of motion.

Use Your Mind and Breath

You'll discover that your mind and your breath are powerful during deep stretches. If you mentally resist the stretch, so will your muscles and tendons. Surrender your mind to the stretch, and your muscles will begin to release. Breathe deeply. On every exhalation, concentrate on unclenching the tight muscles. Picture them releasing, becoming soft and pliant.

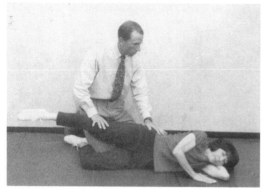

Photo 47. Repeated contractions of right abductors with therapist.

Next, to strengthen the opposite muscle group, the weak abductors, you'll perform **repeated contractions** against resistance offered by the therapist. Starting at your newly established end-range of motion, push hard and fast four times against the therapist's hand, then hold the contraction steady while the therapist counts to four (Photo 47). You'll do this several times until the abductors begin to fatigue. Fatigue causes tissue breakdown, then the muscle rebuilds itself, coming back stronger. The same sustained, passive stretch can be applied to any tight muscles around the hip, and repeated contractions performed to strengthen weak muscles.

Strength Tests

You may decide to visit a physical therapist to see which of your muscles are weak and which are strong. Each body has its own idiosyncrasies: the most common muscular imbalances of hip patients may or may not apply to you.

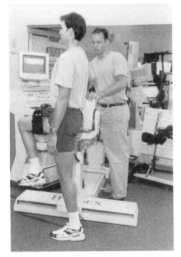

Photo 48. Biodex strength test.

To test the strength in the various muscles surrounding your hip joint, physical therapists either use their hands to perform a manual resistance test or they use machines like Cybex or Biodex (see Photo 48.) All planes of movement are tested: abduction, adduction, flexion, extension, internal rotation, and external rotation. A manual test is obviously subjective, based on the therapist's opinion of how much resistance you can withstand. Such a test might lead your therapist to conclude that both of your hips are reasonably equal in strength. However, an objective test on a Biodex, which computes strength, range of motion, power, and endurance might find subtle differences. The printouts from the machine's computer compare your involved (painful) hip to your uninvolved (healthy) hip so that you can read the difference between the two, read weakness that perhaps had previously gone undetected.

Here's how the Biodex and Cybex work: While most exercise equipment offers dead weight to be lifted by the patient, Biodex and Cybex machines provide **isokinetic exercise,** which means they match the resistance given by the patient. As hard as you push, it pushes back with equal force. This is a safe and efficient way to test the strength of the various muscle groups, because you'll never meet more resistance than you can handle, since the resistance always equals the force applied. The harder your strong muscles push, the more the machine resists. Yet when a weak muscle group is tested, the machine resists with equally weak resistance. If you visit a physical therapist at the beginning of your hip program, ask for a Biodex or Cybex test to establish your baseline. Then retest every month or so to see the progression. Your program can be modified based on your test scores, so you'll always be moving closer to symmetry in both hips in terms of strength, range, power, and endurance.

Although isokinetic machines are normally used strictly for measurement, they can occasionally be used for treatment as well. For example, if you've been in a hip rehab program for a month and have gained overall strength in your painful hip but the Biodex test shows that your right abductors are still weak, you might perform abduction on the Biodex machine for a week or so to chart the improvement of strength in that specific muscle.

Training Muscles in Their Primary Function

Some muscles are primarily movers; others are primarily stabilizers. Your hip flexors and extensors are primarily movers; they move your leg forward and backward. Your external and internal hip rotators are primarily stabilizers; most of the time they work to stabilize your hips. Although your hip abductors and adductors *can* cause movement, most of the time they, too, stabilize your hips. For instance, your abductors work as movers when you lift your leg to the side, but that's a movement seldom performed in daily life. Rather, the abductors primarily keep your pelvis from collapsing with each step as you walk, run, and go about your day: they are primarily stabilizers.

When you strengthen a muscle, you want to exercise it the way it normally functions. Movers should be strengthened with movement exercise while stabilizers should be strengthened with **isometric exercise**—a contraction of the muscle with little or no movement. When you walk, you are exercising the muscles in their correct way: the abductors, adductors, internal rotators, and external rotators stabilize the hips, while the flexors and extensors move the legs forward and backward.

Some exercises shown ask the stabilizers to perform active movement, as in Exercise 20, Lateral Leg Raises (page 101), and Exercise

22, Leg Circles (page 102), for a reason. In those specific exercises you're using the water's buoyancy to increase your hip's range of motion. You're also developing equal strength in the muscles throughout their increased range of motion. When you perform a leg circle in the water, you encounter exactly the same amount of resistance through every curve of that circular movement. You can't create similar isokinetic resistance for the hip on land, so it's important to do that crucial movement in the water.

Some of the land exercises in Chapter 9 at first use active movement to strengthen your abductors, adductors, internal rotators, and external rotators. This is because your muscles are out of balance and require remedial measures. Once you've progressed to the Thera-Band exercises (see page 125), your muscles will be stronger and can work more isometrically against increasing resistance through a narrower range of motion.

Turn to Chapter 9 to begin your land program and move closer to your goal of regaining a normal gait plus full, symmetrical function in everyday life.

9

A Land Program
for Hip Patients

Exercises 1 to 6 are stretching exercises; Exercises 7 to 16 are strengthening exercises. If you do them all on a regular basis, you'll feel the difference in your hip and want to make this program a lifelong habit.

Warm-up Stretches

In all your warm-up stretches, stretch the uninvolved hip first so you can focus on good posture and alignment without the distraction of pain. Stretch to a point of discomfort, then ease off the stretch just a fraction so the stretch will still be challenging, yet you'll be able to hold it for a minute. While you hold the stretch, breathe deeply and try to relax more deeply with every exhalation. Don't push yourself. A slow stretch held for a minute lets gravity do the work for you. Pay careful attention to what is needed from your healthy hip during the stretch so you can apply what you feel to the other side. Then slowly, slowly attempt the stretch on the involved hip, stopping at the point at which you begin to feel pain. Stay there and breathe deeply, monitoring the amount of discomfort you feel. This will lessen over the next weeks, so pay attention. Describe this progress in a rehab journal, or, if you're in a physical therapy program, report to your therapist the changes you feel.

If your hip is fairly limited in its movements, most of these stretches will be difficult at first. Don't be discouraged! Start where you start, and progress from there. Patience and consistency are what count. Your therapist can help you modify the stretch if it's too difficult for you at first.

Establish an exercise space in your home. Chose a specific time to be there and let nothing stop you, short of a hurricane.

> ### Your Rehab Journal
>
> Start a rehab journal and keep it up-to-date. Write down how many sets and reps of the exercises you do each day. Next to that, write down how you feel: Can you stretch further without pain? Do you feel stronger and have less pain during the movements? Are the repetitions easier to do? In a few weeks, refer back to how you felt three to four weeks ago and compare how you feel now. As you record your own progress, you'll become more motivated to continue.

Exercise 1. Hip Flexor Stretch

If you've had knee problems, ask your therapist to guide you through this stretch the first time.

Do this stretch on a rug or padded mat as shown in Photo 49. If you don't have a soft surface, fold a towel under your knee. Place your involved leg forward until your knee is directly over your ankle. Lower your healthy hip downward toward the floor, creating a stretch in the muscles at the front of your uninvolved hip. Breathe deeply and slowly five times. As the muscles relax, lower yourself further. Lift out of the stretch to rest for a moment, then repeat. Then do two reps of this stretch on the involved side.

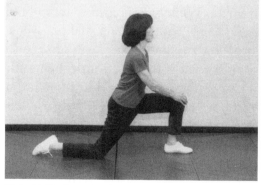

Photo 49. Hip flexor stretch.

Exercise 2. Extensor Stretch

Lie on your back with your legs straight. Keep your head and your lower back flat on the floor throughout this stretch. Clasp your hands under the knee of your uninvolved leg

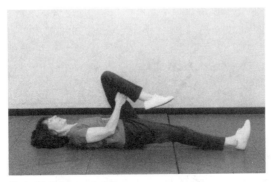

and pull it toward your chest (Photo 50). Breathe slowly and deeply five times. As the muscles relax, try to pull the knee even closer to the chest. Repeat on the involved side. Perform two more Extensor Stretches, one on each side.

Photo 50. Extensor stretch.

Exercise 3. Abductor Stretch

Continue lying on your back. This time, pull your uninvolved leg across your body as shown in Photo 10 on page 7. Your opposite hand is out to the side for balance. Hold this stretch while you breathe deeply and slowly five times. Consciously relax with every exhalation. Come back to the starting position, then perform an abductor stretch on your involved side. Repeat on each side.

Exercise 4. External Rotator Stretch

Continue lying on your back. Bend the knee of the uninvolved leg and place that foot on the floor. Place your other ankle upon that knee and push with your hand to increase the

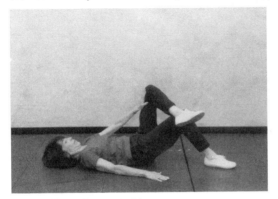

stretch as shown in Photo 51. Hold this stretch for five long slow breaths. Relax, then repeat. Take your time with this stretch. You can't rush the muscles into relaxing. You can allow them to relax only by breathing deeply and being patient. Do the same stretch twice on the other side.

Photo 51. External rotator stretch.

Exercise 5. Internal Rotator Stretch

Sit up with your spine erect and your knees bent to the sides. Put the soles of your feet together with your hands around your ankles (see Photo 11, page 7). Move your feet further or closer to your crotch until you find the most comfortable position. Stay in this position and breathe slowly five times. Relax a few moments, then repeat.

When this becomes easy, use your arms as levers—hold your ankles with your hands and push your knees down with your elbows. Apply the pressure gently to reach your tolerance level.

Exercise 6. Adductor Stretch

Find a wall with enough space for you to assume the position in Photo 52. To reach that position safely, sit sideways with your buttocks touching the wall. Bend your knees and swing your legs upward as you lie back on the floor or mat. If your hamstrings are tight, you may have to stay a foot or so away from the wall to do this stretch. If you have good hamstring flexibility, shift closer so your entire lower body will be touching the wall. Straighten your legs upward and place your hands on the outsides of your thighs. If gravity begins to pull your legs too far apart, use your arms as brakes. Remember to aim toward symmetry. Don't let one leg swing far to the side if the other one is severely limited. Try to keep both legs an equal distance away from the midline of your body.

Stay in this position and breathe deeply at least five times. Come out of this position slowly without making jerky movements. Bend your knees, pull your legs together, and relax a few moments before doing the same stretch again.

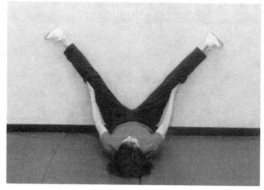

Photo 52. Adductor stretch.

Therapeutic Exercises

In the exercises that follow, you'll be asked to perform a specific number of repetitions of each exercise. After you've completed that first set of reps, rest for up to a minute, then do one or two additional sets as recommended. Pay attention to what you're feeling. Get to know the strengths and weaknesses of each of the muscle groups so your internal monitoring system will become more developed. That way you'll be able to progress intelligently on your own; or you'll be able to provide your therapist with more valuable information. *Do your first set with the uninvolved hip first, then repeat with your involved hip.* Try to duplicate with your involved hip the good movement patterns of your healthy hip. Your goal is to reach equal strength and flexibility in both hips. If you strengthen and stretch one hip, you must also strengthen and stretch the other. Give your healthy hip only a moderate amount of workload to keep it functioning and strong while you work the unhealthy hip to its maximum so it can begin to "catch up" with the healthy hip.

Most people with hip pain have an imbalance in their muscle strength. They usually need to strengthen their extensors and their abductors (see Drawings 4 and 5 on page 12). These are key muscles in stabilizing the pelvis during walking.

Waking Up Your Hip

You may have increased pain at some point during the first few weeks, but don't worry. Nothing's going wrong. You're reactivating something that was lying dormant, so don't let the pain alarm you. Moving your "rusty" hip is like a bear waking from its long winter nap. It yawns and growls and shows its teeth a little before it gets up to resume its life. Continue with the exercises. As you do more of the exercises, you'll start seeing the results. There will be less and less pain and more and more mobility.

Exercise 7. Straight Leg Raise

Lie on your back with your affected leg straight and your unaffected leg bent. Place your hands palms down next to your legs for support. Keep your lower back and both hips in contact with the floor throughout this exercise. Keep your knee straight as you lift your affected leg to the position shown in Photo 12 on page 8, then return it to the floor. Do one set of ten reps on each side, then repeat. When this becomes easy, progress to three sets.

Exercise 8. Hip Abduction

Lie on your side with your unaffected hip up, your body in a straight line. Your head rests on your arm. Don't bend at the hips. Be sure to keep your hips pointed toward the wall in front of you throughout the exercise. Don't let them rotate toward the ceiling. Lift your unaffected leg as high as you can (see Photo 13 on page 8), then slowly return it to the starting position. Do this ten times, then turn on your other side to do a set of ten on your affected side. Repeat so that you've completed two sets of ten on each side. When this becomes easy, do three sets of ten reps.

Exercise 9. Hip Extension

Assume a position on your hands and knees. Keep your back flat, not arched. Now reach your unaffected leg out behind you until your leg is parallel with the floor (see Photo 14 on page 8). Don't lift your leg above this straight position. If this is too difficult for you, lift your leg as high as you can. Hold the position steady while you count to three, then slowly, with control, return your leg to the starting position. Do this ten times, then do a set of ten on the affected side. Go back and forth with sets until you've done two sets of ten reps on each side. When this becomes easy, do three sets of ten reps.

Exercise 10. Adduction with Chair

Find a chair, stool, or coffee table of the proper height for your hip capabilities and set it up so you can place your affected leg on top of the chair. Lie on your side, body straight, with your head resting on your arm. Your unaffected leg rests on the floor. Check to make sure you are not bent at the hips and that your hips and toes are pointed toward the wall in front of you, not angled toward the ceiling. Now lift your bottom leg up to touch the chair (Photo 53). Slowly, with control, lower it to the starting position. Do two sets of ten on this side, resting up to a minute before you change sides, and do two sets of ten reps with the affected leg doing the work. When this becomes easy, do three sets of ten reps.

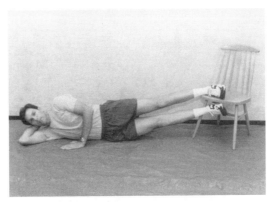

Photo 53. Adduction with chair.

Recovering from implant surgery: Get your surgeon's approval before doing this exercise.

Exercise 11. External and Internal Rotation

Sit in a tall chair or on a tabletop with your knees bent and feet dangling. Perform the exercise with your unaffected leg first. Keep your knee bent and slowly turn your entire leg so the knee points toward the outside (external rotation), as shown in Photo 54, then to the inside (internal rotation), as shown in Photo 55. Start with careful small movements and gradually try to increase the range of your rotations. Each external-internal rotation is one rep. Do one set of ten reps on your unaffected leg, then repeat with your affected leg. Perform one more set of ten reps on each side. Alternate sets between the two sides. After two weeks, increase to 3 sets of 10 reps.

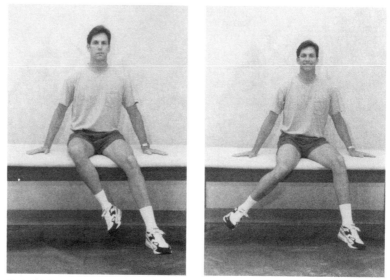

Photo 54. External rotation of right hip.   Photo 55. Internal rotation of right hip.

Recovering from implant surgery: Get your surgeon's permission before doing this exercise.

Dealing with Pain

The first few times you do your exercises, it's probably wise not to take any painkillers prior to the session so that you don't mask your pain and try too hard. However, after you establish your capabilities, you may want to premedicate; that is, you may wish to take some anti-inflammatories prior to doing the work so you can accomplish your tasks more comfortably. If you're seeing a physical therapist, discuss this idea with him or her.

Resistance Exercises with Thera-Bands

Stretchy latex bands can be used to create resistance and increase your workload. Thera-Bands, as they're called, are six inches wide and come in standard colors that designate their graded resistance. Yellow is the easiest to stretch, then red, green, and blue in increasing order of resistance. Extra resistance makes your muscles work harder, and they will quickly gain strength. You'll perform exercises similar to Exercises 7 to 11, but this time you'll be working against gradually increasing resistance.

You'll also have to adjust the band as necessary so you can move through your fullest range of motion without pain. Notice that you'll be standing upright in most of the exercises rather than lying on the floor. If pain in your hip prevents you from standing to do them, stick with Exercises 7 to 11 until you can stand.

As you gain strength each week, you'll progress through the Thera-Bands as shown in Chart A. Move from the yellow to the red Thera-Band only when the exercises become easy and you need more resistance. Use that same criterion moving to green, then blue.

Chart A. Steps in Thera-Band Progression

Yellow:	1 set of 10 reps
	2 sets of 10 reps
	3 sets of 10 reps
Red:	2 sets of 10 reps
	3 sets of 10 reps
Green:	2 sets of 10 reps
	3 sets of 10 reps
Blue:	2 sets of 10 reps
	3 sets of 10 reps

Exercise 12. Straight Leg Raise with Thera-Band

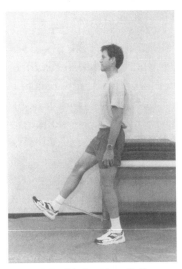

Photo 56. Straight leg raise with Thera-Band.

Tie a knot in your Thera-Band to create a loop. Circle it around the leg of a table and place your unaffected leg in the loop. Stand facing away from the table; if you need to, you can hold on to a chair for balance. Now lift your unaffected leg straight forward as shown in Photo 56. Adjust your position closer to, or further away from, the table as necessary. If you stand too close, there won't be any resistance for the beginning of the exercise. If you stand too far away, you won't be able to lift your leg through the full range of motion. This position may change over a period of weeks, for as you gain strength, you'll be able to pull harder against the band. When you finish one set of ten reps, perform a set with your affected leg. Switch back and forth until you've completed your sets and reps.

Do the number of sets and reps you've mastered. See Chart A, page 123.

Exercise 13. Hip Extension with Thera-Band

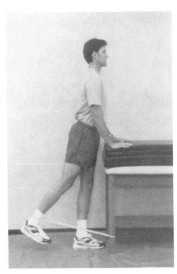

Photo 57. Extension with Thera-Band.

Face the table and place your unaffected leg in the loop. Place your hands on the table for support, then reach your leg straight backward as shown in Photo 57. Adjust your position closer to, or further away from, the table as necessary. Do your first set of ten, then repeat with your affected leg.

Do the number of sets and reps you've mastered. See Chart A, page 123.

Exercise 14. Hip Abduction with Thera-Band

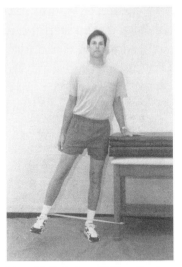

Stand with your side to the table so that your unaffected leg is away from the table and in the Thera-Band. Place your left hand on the table for support, or place a chair in front of you and hold it for balance. Reach your leg to the side as far as you can. If possible, reach all the way to the position shown in Photo 58. Adjust your position to the table depending on what you feel. If it's too easy, move away from the table. If it's too hard, move closer. Just make sure that you have some degree of tension in the band throughout the movement. Complete your first set of ten, then repeat with your affected leg.

Do the number of sets and reps you've mastered. See Chart A, page 123.

Photo 58. Abduction with Thera-Band.

Exercise 15. Hip Adduction with Thera-Band

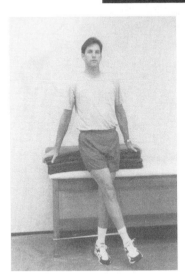

Stand by the table with your unaffected leg inside the Thera-Band. Your legs are directly beneath you in a normal standing position. Place your hands behind you on the table or on a chair in front of you for support. Pull your leg across your body as far as you can, trying to reach the position shown in Photo 59. If this is too difficult for you, move closer to the table to decrease the resistance of the Thera-Band. As you get stronger, move further away. Complete your first set of ten, then repeat with your affected leg.

Do the number of sets and reps you've mastered. See Chart A, page 123.

Recovering from implant surgery: Get your surgeon's approval before doing this exercise.

Photo 59. Adduction with Thera-Band.

Exercise 16. External and Internal Rotation with Thera-Band

Sit on the table with the foot of your unaffected leg inside the Thera-Band. Use your hands to brace yourself as you pull against the Thera-Band so that your foot turns inward and your knee and hip rotate outward (external rotation), as shown in Photo 60. Move the Thera-Band to the other table leg to perform internal rotation as shown in Photo 61. Do all of your sets and reps with your unaffected leg, then repeat on the affected side.

Do the number of sets and reps you've mastered. See Chart A, page 123.

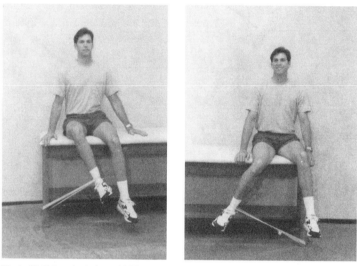

Photo 60. External rotation with Thera-Band.

Photo 61. Internal rotation with Thera-Band.

Recovering from implant surgery: Get your surgeon's approval before doing this exercise.

Remind Yourself to Exercise

To help you remember to do these exercises daily, leave a Thera-Band tied to a table leg or some other appropriate place—a door or a piece of furniture. If it's ready for use, you'll use it.

Apparatus

If you had simply gone to the gym and started using the weight-training equipment right away, you might have done yourself harm. You could have easily overloaded your muscles, tendons, or other soft tissues by asking them to do more than they're capable of, and caused more pain, more tightness, and less mobility. It's necessary to start slowly and increase the workload very gradually over time in order to assure yourself of constant gains without major flare-ups or setbacks. By the time you've worked your way to the blue Thera-Band, you will have developed new strength in your hip and will be functioning better in your daily life.

It may be time to start using weight-training machines that create an ever-increasing workload for the muscles. If you're ready to start this kind of training, a trainer or therapist can show you this new equipment. The weight room offers you a variety of exercises that continue to strengthen all the muscles you've been working. Remember that your goal is to help your weak hip catch up with the healthy hip. Thus you'll challenge the weaker one to its maximum while you let the stronger one work at a more moderate level.

If you don't have an affinity for apparatus, or don't like the idea of training in a gym or health club, you can continue doing three sets of ten reps with the blue Thera-Band at home. Whatever you decide, know that these exercises are now part of your life.

10

Nonsurgical and Surgical Solutions

When you began reading this book, your hip hurt and you didn't know what to do about it.

That must seem like a long time ago, for by now many of you have earned a solution to your problem. Rather than sitting idly by, watching the deterioration of your hip, you followed the advice in the previous chapters: you helped your doctor make a diagnosis; you lost weight; you exercised at home or joined a yoga class. Or you plunged straight into the water for a pool program. Whatever your original degree of hip limitation and pain, you've worked toward a "cure." If nothing else, you've achieved the peace of mind that comes with knowledge.

Some of you will never be concerned about your hip again.

Others, in spite of joint deterioration, are doing fine by wisely managing the soft tissues around your hip joint. You've reduced pain, regained strength, restored lost function and mobility. Although your X ray hasn't changed, you've prevented surgery.

Consider the story of a forty-seven-year-old man who, literally overnight, developed pain in both hips. His orthopedic surgeon took X rays and MRIs and told him he needed implant surgery. By his own acknowledgment this patient had been a couch potato for ten years preceding the diagnosis. He'd lost strength and flexibility from inactivity, so to prepare for surgery he followed the pool program in Chapter

7 twice a week for eight weeks. At the end of that time he was walking without his cane, with no pain in either hip.

By exercising, he had rejuvenated the blood vessels to his muscles and improved his muscle tone. Exercise had caused a hormonal cascade: chemicals stimulated the body to make blood vessels, which increased blood supply to the hip. The collapsed cartilage and bone didn't grow back. Absolutely not! But the patient earned himself a reprieve from surgery. He bought time. If his hips trouble him again in six months or in a year or two, if the pool program doesn't work for him the next time, then he can consult his surgeon and reschedule the operation. It's not uncommon for a hip implant patient to have several such surgeries in a lifetime, so the longer he can put off the first one, the less likely he'll need the second.

Despite your best efforts, however, your pain may continue, and your mobility may worsen. Your orthopedic doctor may offer one last chance to prevent a hip implant: you may be a candidate for the minimally invasive procedure, arthroscopy, a discussion of which follows in Chapter 11.

However, if advanced architectural changes have taken place in your hip joint—a misshapen ball meeting an irregularly shaped socket, no joint space, no cartilage to save—the degenerative process has gone too far for any solution other than a hip implant. Chapter 12 describes this surgery.

Rehab or Prehab?

Regardless of your outcome to date, you should regularly continue your pool and land exercises. If they were a rehab solution to your hip problem that prevented surgery, congratulations! They taught you how to maintain strength, flexibility, and function in your hip, and will be your tool to use for a lifetime.

But even if these exercises didn't prevent surgery, consider them *prehab,* a rehabilitation program to get you in shape prior to surgery. Many patients routinely participate in prehab programs to better help their bodies cope with the stresses of surgery. The fitter you enter the operation room, the quicker you'll return to your sports and daily activities.

11

Hip Arthroscopy

To a certain extent, everything you have learned so far about diagnosing your hip is secondhand information. All the tests, X rays, MRIs, CT Scans, blood work, physical exams, and patient history are like hearing about a friend from another friend. The only true firsthand information comes from looking inside the joint. There I can see exactly what damage may exist: the depth of blemishes on the cartilage, the amount of inflamed synovium, the extent of the tear in the labrum, or the amount of exposed bone. I can then confirm, refine, or reject my earlier diagnosis and, in the same surgical procedure, treat my patient's problem hip.

Arthros in Latin means "joint," and *scope* means "to look inside." During hip arthroscopy I make a tiny puncture wound and insert a pencil-sized optical device into the hip joint. A miniature television camera attached to the arthroscope allows me to view the interior of the joint on a large video monitor.

Before arthroscopic procedures became available on the hip joint, traumatic open procedures were necessary to see inside the joint. Those open procedures meant cutting through the skin and the underlying tissues and dislocating the joint. But now, using the tiny instruments that let me see through a small puncture wound, I can easily get past those same structures: the skin, the muscles, the **subcutaneous** tissues, the subcutaneous fat, the ligaments, and the joint capsule. These days, a view inside the joint to obtain firsthand information isn't nearly so costly in terms of tissue damage.

A Case History of Arthroscopic Diagnosis

I recently scoped a young woman whose hip had been tender for more than six months. There was no history of trauma to the joint and no infection. She was thirty-one years old. She had had blood tests for various rheumatological diseases, but all had come back negative, so we decided to look through the scope to make a diagnosis.

I saw an unbelievable amount of inflammation in the lining of the joint, as if I were looking into a cave roofed with stalagmites and stalactites. Those points of inflammation, called **fronds,** were hanging from the ceiling of the joint, creating the swelling and ultimately working on the destruction of the joint. I sensed immediately this was rheumatoid arthritis and sent a specimen of the joint lining to the lab. In this way, the arthroscopy and the pathologist confirmed a diagnosis of rheumatoid arthritis.

Although RA is a systemic disease, it had selected this particular hip for its starting point. The young woman thought she had only a hip problem, but she found instead the beginning of a lifelong problem. The correct diagnosis, however, will allow her rheumatologist to use more aggressive medication and physical therapy. These treatments may help her postpone or prevent surgery in her hip and other joints.

Lavage

When the scope is first inserted into the joint, I can see little because the acidic, deteriorated joint fluid is clouding my vision. As I perform the arthroscopy, I pump clear salt water into the joint both to clear the vision and to flush out the old, destructive joint fluid, a process equivalent to changing the oil in a car. In a car, the dirty oil that causes damage to the car's engine is replaced by a clear yellow liquid. In the human body, the joint's synovial fluid that is thick and debris-laden is replaced by harmless sterile salt water.

This cleansing of a joint is called **lavage,** and it offers the arthritic joint a respite from its troubles.

My goal in a hip arthroscopy is to clean up both the joint's structure and its fluids. We believe people get better not only from removing any rough edges that scrape and damage the cartilage, but also because of the lavage.

Temporary or Permanent Solutions

Some conditions can be partially or fully resolved with arthroscopy. They are:

Degenerative arthritis
Loose bodies or fragments in the joint
A torn labrum
Synovitis

Degenerative Arthritis

Let's look at arthritis in phases. You start with a normal joint—then something goes wrong. In Phase 1 you have pain, extra fluid in the joint, and swelling in the lining. Still, you have, essentially, a normal joint.

In Phase 2 there is increased pain. The muscles around the hip start shutting down; stiffness creeps into the joint and the capsule thickens. Doctors are not sure which happens first, but the abnormal internal fluid appears about the time that the smooth glistening cartilage starts to have cracks or fissures in it. The cracks that start as razor cuts start widening and getting deeper, becoming injuries to the cartilage.

During Phase 3 a piece of the cartilage lifts off from one of the deeper and wider cracks. It is probably still hinged at its base, but that cracked piece, a flap, is starting to develop.

In Phase 4, the flap that lifted breaks off and leaves behind a hole, a defect in the cartilage surface. That piece of cartilage is nourished by the joint fluid, so even though it is no longer attached to anything, it isn't going to die. It will grow bigger and may even calcify. Phases 1 through 3 show early arthritic changes in the joint with deepening cracks in the cartilage. Phase 4 is the final stage, where exposed bone is showing through the damaged cartilage. Arthroscopy can be appropriate for Phases 1 through 3, but an implant would be needed by the time Phase 4 has been reached.

Loose Bodies

Healthy cartilage has a smooth, billiard ball–like surface. As degenerative arthritis progresses, turning that smooth surface into a cracking surface, some of the cracks break off and float loosely, unattached in the joint. Those fragments are called loose bodies, and they become an annoyance that leads to trouble. They can cause a "catching" in the joint. They can also scratch and damage the smooth areas of the joint, so I like to remove them as soon as they are identified before they can ruin what might otherwise still be a fairly good hip joint.

Before arthroscopy became available for the hip joint, people had to live with loose bodies in their hip joints until the pain or limitation became such that they warranted removal through an open procedure.

Torn Labrum

The labrum is a rim of **fibrocartilage** that runs completely around the acetabulum (the socket side of the hip joint), effectively deepening the socket and increasing the "capture" of the socket onto the ball. (See Drawing 2, page 10.)

I believe that the labrum may be one of the causes for arthritic deterioration of the hip. If a labrum tears and flips into the joint, it starts to scratch the surface. If I can trim that frayed labrum out before it acts like sandpaper and scratches a hole through the surface of the cartilage, I may be able to stop a hip's deterioration even before it begins.

If your hip pops or locks (freezes in position), you may have a torn labrum. If I see a frayed labrum through the scope, I remove the torn part and often see an improvement of the hip's function. The hip is a very secure joint; removing some of the labrum won't make the joint unstable.

Synovitis

When the synovial lining of the hip joint is so inflamed that it causes disabling pain, we consider removing the inflamed tissue. A complete **synovectomy** (removal of the synovial lining) isn't possible through the arthroscope, but when the portions of the synovium that can be reached with the scope are removed, a patient will feel significant improvement.

Arthroscopy and Exercise:
Two Case Histories of Solutions

One of my arthroscopy patients had been a professional dancer from the time he was fifteen years old. When he was twenty-two, he began having deep pain in his left hip. Twice he had cortisone injections in his hip, but the shots failed to help. He was in nonstop pain but developed ways to cope with it: he iced, he stretched, and he was able to perform on stage, but the pain in his hip was constant. It didn't get better, and it didn't get worse.

At twenty-four, he made a transition from performer to massage therapist for the Royal Danish Ballet, but even when he stopped dancing, the pain didn't go away. He decided to research the treatment options for his hip. He moved to Los Angeles and heard about the arthroscopic hip surgery I was starting to do. I was very optimistic after I examined him and studied his X rays. I explained that we could probably eliminate his pain and improve the mobility of his hip. But first we both wanted to see if the pool program might help him avoid surgery altogether. After six weeks in the pool, he had improved his strength and flexibility, but the deep pain was still present.

We did the arthroscopy and found perfect cartilage but inflamed synovial lining. We debulked the synovium and washed out the corrosive joint fluid and left him with a clean hip joint. Within a few days after the arthroscopy, he had no pain whatsoever. He even went hiking three days after surgery and was back in the pool in a week. His rehab went very quickly as he regained strength, flexibility, and function in the pool. He reports that he hasn't had any problems with his hip since surgery (see Photo 62), and I don't expect him to. He'll probably never need implant surgery.

Another patient was a fifty-eight-year-old former professional basketball player. He developed a hip flexor muscle contracture such that he could no longer fully straighten his hip, and his buttocks muscles had severely atrophied. His cartilage,

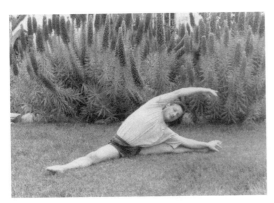

Photo 62. Hip arthroscopy patient stretching.

however, still looked good on the X ray, so I did the arthroscopy to clean out his sore joint. Once the inflammation was vacuumed out, I saw glistening, smooth cartilage. He was in the pool almost every day for months after that surgery and regained lost motion and strength in that hip. Now, four years later, his intention is not to have implant surgery but to continue with his exercise regimen to keep his own hip.

I want to emphasize that it wasn't just the arthroscopic surgery that helped these patients get better; it was the surgery in partnership with the exercise programs.

Buying Time

An arthroscopy may be able to solve your hip problem for a year, two years, a decade, or even for good. For a few lucky patients it can mean the end of hip problems altogether, but for the majority of people with progressive arthritis in a hip, it usually serves as a way to "buy time" before the more serious hip implant surgery becomes necessary. The implant operation is an end-stage procedure to salvage your hip. You don't want to go to that stage yet if you don't absolutely have to. In fact, you don't really want to do *any* surgery unless pain or lack of function is decreasing the quality of your life.

A Case History of Buying Time

A pilot living in California was also a serious beach volleyball competitor. About the time he turned forty, he began getting a jab of pain in his right hip when he first stood after sitting during a long flight. The pain would then subside as he walked through the airport after landing. Over the next few months his hip grew progressively worse. He asked his doctor friends for advice, researched his condition on the Internet, and within a year came to my office. His X rays confirmed that his hip condition was osteoarthritis. The sharp starting pain he had was predictable and stable, but he was now also getting shooting nerve pain emanating from the groin.

To make sure that his pain wasn't referred pain from a pinched nerve in his back, we did a lidocaine injection into the hip joint. Although we found spurs and degenerative disks in his lower back, most of the pain he felt in his leg and hip was coming from the arthritic process in his hip. He had enough cartilage to warrant doing an arthroscopy. His pain wasn't debilitating, but he decided to be aggressive. He understood that the surgery would clean out his deteriorating joint and give him a chance to do some advanced pool therapy to regain his full range of motion and become as pain-free as possible.

Ten days after the arthroscopy he was in the pool, and within a month he had regained nearly complete range of motion in his hip, although he continued to have mild discomfort. From what I saw through the scope, his long-range prognosis is not as good as the Danish dancer's. This pilot may need an implant some years from now. To delay that as long as possible, he has cut back his workouts and recreational activities by more than half. He's learned he can occasionally play tennis, paddle tennis, and volleyball. He can take long hikes and even downhill ski. But those activities have to be just that, *occasional.* The staple of his fitness routine is mountain biking, weight training, and the pool. He ices, stretches, and gets to the pool religiously. Those are the things that keep his hip running smoothly in spite of arthritis.

Now, four years after the arthroscopy, he says his hip is better than before surgery. He gets Deep-tissue massage when he feels particularly stiff, and he tries other remedies as he learns about them. His change in lifestyle, combined with the arthroscopy, may have bought him at least a decade or more before considering implant surgery.

Hope for the Future

Recently I read that researchers have begun injecting hyaluronic acid into knee joints to enhance the quality of the hyaline cartilage. The hope is that the arthritis-damaged cartilage will utilize new building blocks injected into the joint to repair itself. The future treatment for arthritic hips may also lie in this direction. I'm optimistic this might be a realistic way to prevent implant surgery in the future.

—*Robert Klapper, M.D.*

Are You a Candidate for Hip Arthroscopy?

Many patients suffer from degenerative arthritis of the hip, but only a small percentage are candidates for arthroscopy. Although there aren't any fixed criteria for what makes an ideal candidate, with my patients I look at the following:

- Have you diligently tried the pool and land programs for at least three months and not found relief from your symptoms? Before I consider any surgery, no matter how minimally invasive it may be, I want to see if it's possible for you to regain strength, flexibility, and function through exercise. If you tell me you made an honest effort and failed, I'll consider performing an arthroscopy if the other criteria also support that.
- What is your age? Generally speaking, the younger you are, the more likely I'll consider doing an arthroscopy to try to preserve the hip as long as possible and delay any need for hip implant surgery.
- How long have you been having symptoms? Even if you are older, I might consider doing an arthroscopy if the symptoms have just begun and I think I can buy enough time that your hip might see you through the rest of your life without implant surgery.
- What does the X ray look like? The X ray should show only *mild* changes of arthritis. We both have to keep in mind, though, that what the X ray shows us and what I'll actually see looking through the scope may be two different things. We may see a fine preservation of joint space on the X ray, yet discover during arthroscopy that the surface of the articular cartilage is fairly damaged.

My goal as a surgeon is to maximize whatever can be kept intact for each patient, so I'm willing to enter the operating room not knowing whether an arthroscopy will be enough to help the patient or whether I'll have to do implant surgery. I ask the patient to be prepared to go either way. Patients in this situation donate two units of blood as if we were going to do the implant surgery, even though we may not. Not every orthopedic surgeon is willing to be put in this position, but sometimes there is not enough information for a definitive decision until I've taken a look through the scope.

Hip Arthroscopic Surgery

If you are a good candidate for hip arthroscopy and have found a surgeon, you'll want to ask him or her what to expect throughout your day in the hospital.

For now I'll be your guide. On the day of surgery you'll pass through admissions and **pre-op** and be taken into the operating room (OR) by the nurses and the anesthesiologist. You have probably decided which kind of anesthesia to use—an epidural, a spinal, or a general, and your doctor will confirm your choice with the anesthesiologist, who then administers it. Then you'll be given **intravenous (IV)** antibiotics to guard against infection. The leg that is to be scoped is treated with an antiseptic solution and draped so that only the area of the hip joint and the leg involved is exposed. The rest of the body is covered.

Your doctor will use special instruments that allow him to make a path through the tissues into the joint in as gentle a way as possible. When he first gets inside the joint, he won't be able to see much, because the synovium will block his vision. He will start cutting it away and vacuuming it out. Once he's cleaned away enough of this inflamed material, there will be more visibility. With the synovium trimmed back, the ball, the cartilage, the capsule, the labrum, and any loose bodies inside the joint become visible so he can work on them.

Once he's cleaned out all the inflamed tissues, removed all the loose bodies, and smoothed down all the rough edges, he will remove the instruments and the arthroscope. The two puncture wounds are closed with one stitch for each puncture site. A sterile compressive dressing will be placed over the hip, and you'll be taken to the recovery room.

Although you will be in the OR only half an hour, you will spend the same length of time in the recovery room as any other patient following more major surgery, because your anesthesia has to wear off. If you need pain medication, it will be administered. You'll most likely go home the same day.

You will want to do everything you can to prevent any sort of surgery, even arthroscopy, a minimally invasive procedure. But if you do need it, you should talk to your surgeon about the risks that accompany this and every surgical procedure.

Recovery from Arthroscopy

Research has shown that proper use of exercise speeds healing and that lack of exercise during the early stages of rehabilitation may result in permanent disability. You need to move, but use comfort as your guide.

You will be offered crutches for comfort and can either use them or not, as needed. Although you can get up and walk around immediately, you'll be encouraged to take it easy for a few days. You may be given a cooling unit to take home, which works just like ice packs around the surgical site. After a few days you'll return to your doctor's office to change the bandage.

You can do the land exercises gently (Exercises 1 to 11, pages 118 to 124) as soon as your pain tolerance allows. About a week after surgery, the stitches will be removed, and a day or two later, you can get in the pool with *no restrictions whatsoever*. Take your hip through its complete range of motion if possible; if you experience pain, work only to your level of tolerance.

A Window of Opportunity Following Arthroscopy

After a hip arthroscopy, you should feel significantly better within a week or two. The inflamed tissues and destructive fluids have been removed—your pain should be greatly reduced.

Now you need to work the joint so it can become as healthy as possible during the brief window of opportunity: now, while your hip is free from pain, you should do the pool and land programs to make the muscles stronger around the joint before your body is able to recreate the corrosive enzymes in the joint fluid again.

This is the time to force the joint to become more limber and to achieve its healthy range of motion so you can reverse the vicious cycle of loss of function. The stronger your muscles, the more they can act like springs or shock absorbers for your hip and the less the weight-bearing surfaces inside the joint will pound upon each other. Then, when the arthritic process in your hip begins to create corrosive joint fluid again, you'll be able to fight back with muscular strength and flexibility. Ultimately, you may need further surgery, but arthroscopy can serve as a stopgap measure to keep you functioning for years without major surgery.

Use your window of opportunity wisely.

12

Hip Implant Surgery

This is the chapter we hoped you wouldn't have to read!

It is intended as an overview for patients who have put forth serious effort in a pool or land therapy program but who believe they have failed in making any improvement in their hip's condition. They are probably taking pain medication, but their discomfort continues to wake them in the night. They may even have consulted a surgeon and been told that an arthroscopic procedure would be unlikely to give them relief. They have reached the point at which, because of pain, they can neither face their daily physical activities nor sleep through the night.

If you are one of these patients, you'll find that knowing what takes place during implant surgery will make the operation less frightening to contemplate.

More Hope for the Future

Technological advances continue to offer new hope and more options for people with hip problems, offering one more reason to try to postpone surgery. We *all* hope for a more elegant and holistic approach to solving hip problems, and every day brings us closer to it. It's possible that in five or ten years we might not be doing hip implant surgery. There may be a laser procedure that's appropriate. Even further into the future, gene therapy may eliminate many hip conditions, and the most likely technique to be used in the future is the injection of cartilage-enhancing substances directly into the hip joint.

Although I perform surgery in the operating room (OR) at Cedars-Sinai Hospital in Los Angeles, you can be assured that this hospital will be very similar to the hospital you'll be going to in Phoenix, Miami, New York, or anywhere else in the United States.

Now let me be your surgeon for a chapter.

Positioning the Patient

You'll be wheeled into the OR lying on your back. If you've been given a general anesthesia, you most likely won't remember these events. The anesthesiologist stands at the head of the table. He administers the anesthesia and monitors your vital signs throughout the surgery. The surgical equipment is at the opposite end of the room. Once the anesthetic has taken full effect, we position the patient for surgery. Your surgeon may do things differently, but the hip surgery I do requires that the patient be placed on his side. We gently turn him so that the hip needing surgery is up. It's important for me to position my own patients rather than have the assistants do it for me, because I want to make sure the patient isn't leaning one way or the other. We hold the patient in place with positioners on the OR table. These padded bumpers keep the patient in a fixed "home base" position so that while we're moving the leg during surgery, the pelvis and the rest of the body will remain stable.

Shaving, Sterilizing, and Dressing the Leg

If you have a fair amount of hair on your body, we shave the area where I'll be making the incision. The nurse uses an antiseptic solution to sterilize the entire leg. Even the toes are covered with antiseptic. Various drapes are placed so that your full body is covered. Next we wrap sterile dressings around the leg up to the site of the incision. This is an extra effort to minimize bacterial exposure of the wound. We want everything covered except the surgical site.

The Incision

I use a felt-tip marker to draw a line where I'm going to make the incision (Photo 63). The line for this patient is approximately eight inches long and angled back into the buttocks, but if you have more fat below your skin, the incision will be longer. The cross marks help me close the wound correctly at the end of surgery. Without cross marks, it would be more difficult to line up the two ends of the wound— there could be a puckering or unevenness to the closure, as if you buttoned your shirt one button off.

Notice the clear plastic that's placed over the skin in the area of the incision. This is to sterilize further the site of the incision.

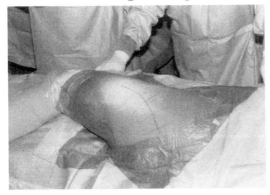

Photo 63. Dr. Klapper draws a line where he will make the incision.

Surgery

Although you'll commonly hear this operation called a "total hip replacement," I am *not* totally replacing your hip. I'm resurfacing the two sides of the joint, putting in new pieces to take the place of your faulty cartilage. My goal is to reproduce a frictionless surface on both sides of the joint.

When I've opened the hip joint, I carefully measure the dimensions of the ball so I know exactly what to replace. I remove the defective cartilage and the underlying bone, which means removing the entire head of the femur. (Photo 64 shows the pits and craters in the cartilage that ruined the smooth functioning of this hip.)

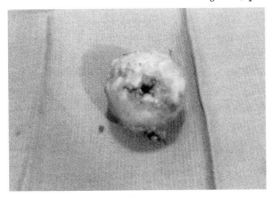

Photo 64. The defective, pitted ball (head of the femur) is removed.

Next I prepare the shaft of the femur to accept the new implant. I create a tunnel in the soft marrow inside the bone that will match the shape of the implant, then put the implant snugly into place. On the socket side of the joint, I again take careful measurements before I start so we can recreate the same dimensions. I use what looks like a dome-shaped cheese grater to remove a potato-chip thickness of the cartilage from inside the socket. Then I prepare the bony bed to receive the new socket. The X ray in Figure 7 shows what the hip looks like after surgery, with both pieces in place.

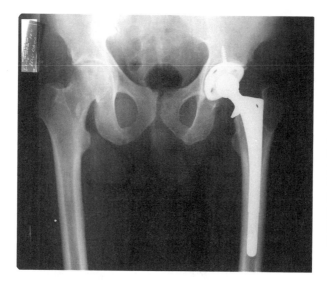

Figure 7. Implant X ray. On the left is a normal hip with an intact joint space and preservation of the ball. On the right, you can see the implant, which reveals a new surface to both the ball and the socket sides of the joint. Notice that the implant sits fully within the walls of the femur. No cement is used to hold either of these implants in place, although a single screw in the pelvis prevents the socket from rotating while bone grows into it.

Custom-Making Your Implant

Not long ago, we had only small, medium, and large implants, and the surgeon had to chip away the patient's bone to fit the implant. Now we fit the patient's bone exactly. We use tools to measure inside the bone at the time of surgery. Thus we can create the perfect-sized implant for a basketball player who's seven feet tall as well as a jockey who's five feet tall—and it's all done during the surgery. Because the pieces of the implant come in various lengths, widths, and sizes, we're able to fit them together in various combinations, creating a large number of options.

During surgery, while I'm taking a firsthand look at the quality of the bone, I can also make the decision about whether to use cement to hold the implant in place or whether the bone is healthy enough to grow into a porous-coated implant.

The implant consists of the following pieces:

The ball. There are different ball sizes since this is the main place where I adjust the leg length. Ball size #1 versus ball size #4 can provide an extra inch in the overall length of the leg.

The implant. The implant is the metal alloy piece that fits into the shaft of your femur. It comes in various widths and lengths, so a correct size can be chosen to create the right implant to fit your bone. The ball fits onto the end of the implant, in effect becoming the new head of your femur.

The socket. We also have different sizes and choices for the socket side of the joint. There are smooth sockets that require cement to fix them to the bone as well as sockets with multiple holes and a roughened surface that allows the bone to grow into them.

By carefully choosing each of the three pieces of the implant and judging the quality of the bone, we're able to build for each individual the most durable, efficient new hip joint possible.

Closing the Incision

When the surgical work is complete, we immediately begin closing the wound using sutures to bring the various deep tissues together. Once we reach the skin, however, we use staples to pinch the skin together. The cross marks (shown in Photo 63 on page 147) guide us so we can precisely restore the dimensions to both sides of the incision.

When Surgery Is Over

The patient is gently returned to a position lying on his back. Inflatable stockings are placed around both of his legs and a pillow is strapped

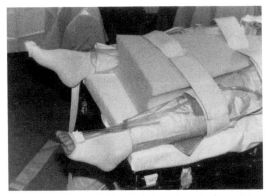

Photo 65. Inflatable stockings and abduction pillow are put in place before the patient is transferred out of the operating room.

between his legs to keep them apart (Photo 65). You'll learn more about the stockings and the pillow in Chapter 13.

Even though I do everything in my power to help my patients prevent or delay surgery for as long as possible, when it's time for the hip implant, I encourage them to look forward to an improved quality of life. Hip surgery is one of the reasons I'm so passionate about orthopedics, because I'm taking one of the most debilitating, life-interrupting problems that can happen to people, and giving them their lives back.

13

In and Out of the Hospital

If you've never had an operation, or never spent time in a hospital, you'll have dozens of questions, concerns, and, yes, fears as you prepare for hip implant surgery. In this chapter we'll try to allay your fears and concerns by giving you so much information that you'll feel like a veteran on arrival at the hospital.

One of the first things you can do is talk directly to another of your surgeon's patients who has successfully gone through the whole process. I make that easy in my office by having a list of patients who are good at talking about what happened to them. I've got a range of ages and personality types on the list, so if I have a patient who is an active woman in her forties who wants to return to skiing, I look at my list and match her up with someone with similar concerns and goals. I match women with women and men with men, and I do my best to match their diagnoses exactly. If you have a fracture, arthritis, a congenital problem, or an additional back problem, you should speak to someone else with the same condition who has gone through the same surgery.

A patient may have questions she isn't comfortable discussing with me, such as "When can I get up by myself to go to the bathroom again?" or "When can I have sex again?" It's also important for patients to ask such questions as "Am I going to be able to reach my doctor by phone after surgery?" "Is his or her bedside manner genuine?" "What was your relationship like with the doctor in terms of care before, during, and after the surgery?" Talking these things over with an "experienced" patient can give you valuable information and reassurance.

Prior to Surgery

Between the time your surgery is scheduled and the date of the surgery itself, there are several things you can do to help ensure the best possible outcome.

Donate Blood

There's no question that the safest blood to receive if you lose blood during surgery is your own. That's why you'll want to donate blood designated for your own use prior to surgery. In my practice, two pints is the usual number, but check with your doctor. Family members might want to donate blood for you, which is admirable, but even if they're the most clean-living people you know, they may have picked up something unbeknownst to them just by eating in a restaurant. The big worry with blood transfusions, of course, is HIV, but you could also be exposed to hepatitis or other infectious diseases from someone else's blood.

Talk to your surgeon about the issue of donating blood, then find out which blood bank works with your hospital and contact it. A transfusion specialist will see you and go over the details. Generally the blood can be stored for about six weeks before surgery. I tell my patients that once they pick a surgical date, they can count back from that date. Give a pint of blood, wait a week, rest, give a second pint of blood, wait a week, rest, and then have the surgery. In a time that can be filled with anxiety, it's good to do things in a smooth, orchestrated fashion.

Visit an Internist or Your Family Doctor

Although internists, family practice doctors, and general practitioner doctors are slightly different, all three of them look at your overall medical condition. About a week before your scheduled operation, you'll have a general physical exam to make sure that you're a safe candidate for surgery. The doctor will test your heart and lungs and take blood tests and a chest X ray. All of these pre-op tests make sure you're fit for the surgery.

If you don't have your own medical doctor, or if your doctor doesn't practice at your surgeon's hospital, your surgeon should recommend one for you.

Take a Pre-op Education Class

Not all hospitals have a pre-op education class. If yours doesn't, you'll actually get a miniversion of such a class right here in this chapter, a comprehensive preview of what's to come. If your hospital *does* have a pre-op class, you'll most likely meet a surgical nurse and a physical therapist who will talk you through your entire stay in the hospital. You'll learn about anesthesia, painkillers, and the use of walkers and crutches. The hip precautions (see page 163) will be discussed to prepare you for the coming restrictions in your movements.

Research shows that patients who attend a presurgical education class are discharged from the hospital sooner than those who do not attend. They know what to expect, so they handle it better—and that includes handling pain. The class also helps eliminate the shock some patients experience when they're asked to get out of bed so quickly after surgery. If they're unprepared by such a class, some of them will say, "What do you mean I have to get up the very next day?" Research shows patients have to get upright almost immediately for improved recovery.

Prepare Your Home for Your Return

Especially if you live alone, you must have your things prepared in advance. Think about what things you have to bend over for in your daily life. Move them to a higher position. If your chairs are low, pile one cushion onto another to give you height. You'll want to sit high, with your hip bent less than 90 degrees for the first six weeks.

Consider having meals already prepared and in your freezer, and groceries in your cupboards. Move comfortable clothes to the front of your closets.

Understand Your Insurance Benefits

During your stay in the hospital, you'll want to devote your time and effort to healing. This means you should do all the research about your insurance well before your operation.

Many of today's health plans use various "networks," groups of health care providers that contract with your hospital. Your surgeon and the hospital you choose may both be part of your network, but many of the services they'll use are not. The **anesthesiologist** is a medical doctor who administers and supervises the **anesthesia,** the drugs that will sedate you or make you unconscious. The anesthesiologist who usually works in the operating room with your surgeon might not be part of your network. The lab that does your urine and blood work might not be either. If you go blindly into surgery without researching, you'll receive bills from companies you've never heard of after the surgery. Many of them won't be part of your network and that will trigger a different, and probably higher, deductible on your insurance.

You should take the time to find out exactly what services you'll need for the surgery and what companies you can select that are part of your network. This can save you hundreds of dollars. You may, however, decide to keep your doctor's "team" together. For instance, if the anesthesiologist who usually works with your surgeon in the operating room isn't in your network, you may decide that their close working relationship is worth the extra money.

In particular, you should know what your post-hospital benefits are. Does your insurance pay for home care or another extended care facility? Your doctor wants you well taken care of, and he might say, "Since you don't have anyone at home to help, we'll send you to this place." But your insurance may not pay for the place he has in mind.

Find out what equipment your insurance will pay for. In your room, you'll use a high toilet seat for comfort and safety, and you'll be given one to take home as well. The physical therapists will teach you how to use crutches or a walker safely. You'll continue to need those crutches or the walker when you first leave the hospital. The occupational therapist will teach you to use a reaching device so you won't have to bend over to pick things up from the floor. The therapists will teach you tricks using this "reacher" so you can safely put on your shoes and socks or pick up things you drop. The hospital staff will do their best to verify what will be paid for by your insurance, but you should know, too. If they send you home with equipment that won't be paid for by your insurance, you will be paying for it.

Day of Surgery: Check-in

Most patients are asked to check into the hospital the day of surgery, two hours before the scheduled time of the operation. Operating rooms generally open around 7:30 A.M., so your arrival time might be quite early. You should find out about parking in advance. You don't want to be late because you couldn't find a parking place.

Wear casual, loose-fitting clothing that won't press against your incision site on your return home. Wear a comfortable pair of shoes that you can slip into easily without bending to put them on.

You'll start at the admissions office. The admissions desk will have a list of all the people who are having surgery that day, so they'll be expecting you. Study the following checklist. Then when you talk to that other patient who's had surgery similar to yours, ask if there was anything unique about your particular hospital. Was there anything he or she forgot to bring from home that would have made the hospital stay more pleasant?

Checklist: What to Take to the Hospital
- A list of the medications you're currently taking and the amount you take daily of each. Don't bring the actual medications with you. The hospital will supply them for you.
- Pajamas, a robe, slippers, glasses, hearing aid, dentures, and personal toiletries such as your toothbrush, hairbrush, shampoo, and deodorant.
- Insurance information.
- Emergency phone numbers.
- Your cane, crutches, or walker, if you use them. Label them with your name. If they're misplaced while you're in surgery, they can easily be returned to you.

- A copy of your advance directives. These are written statements such as a living will or health care power of attorney. They communicate your wishes for your health care if you are unable to communicate those wishes for yourself. Advance directives forms are usually available through your hospital.
- Don't bring anything of value into the hospital the day of surgery. You don't want to lose something you cherish.
- Bring only a few dollars in cash. Don't bring credit cards with you.
- Leave all jewelry at home.

If You Check into the Hospital Alone

A growing number of patients don't live with family members and are therefore responsible for their own health care, even during the difficult days of surgery. Many questions and logistical challenges will present themselves, so we've offered some suggestions.

- Bring a *copy* of your driver's license and insurance card with you when you check in, not the actual documents.
- Take a taxi or have a friend drop you off at the hospital, since you won't be able to drive yourself home.
- Try to make arrangements for a friend or neighbor to bring your favorite bathrobe, pajamas, shorts, or other necessities on the second or third day. You'll be wearing a hospital gown the first day or two.
- Leave your favorite wristwatch at home. But some rooms don't have clocks, so you may want to bring an inexpensive wristwatch.

Day of Surgery: Admission

A hospital employee or volunteer will take you to your next stop, a room in which you prepare for surgery. A nurse will admit you and review any requests your surgeon may have made.

At this point you will change into your hospital gown. It will button or tie in the back. Your clothes will be placed in a bag. If someone is with you, this is when you'll give them all your belongings, including your wristwatch, rings, and other jewelry that you forgot to leave at home. If you're alone, your bag will be locked in a special closet until you've arrived in your room after surgery. Later that day these belongings will be brought to you.

Now that you're in your hospital gown, you'll wait until the surgical staff is ready for you. One of the reasons you're asked to be at the hospital two hours prior to your surgery is that if someone else's surgery is cancelled at the last minute, you could be whisked off into the operating room (OR) early. On the other hand, an operation might take longer than was expected, and you could go into surgery late. The timing of your surgery depends on what happens to the patients in your designated operating room. More than one surgeon may be sharing the room that day, so the timing doesn't always depend on your doctor alone. When it's time, you'll be taken to the pre-op holding area and your family will be shown to the waiting room.

Day of Surgery: The Pre-op Holding Room

A hospital employee will pick you up approximately forty-five minutes before your surgery is expected to begin. You'll be taken by wheelchair to pre-op, a holding room near the operating room. There the surgical staff will settle you onto a gurney (a stretcher on wheels) and make final preparations for surgery. The nurses in the pre-op room will introduce themselves. They'll always tell you what they're going to do before they do it.

If you wear glasses, contact lenses, a hearing aid, or dentures, you'll keep all of these in place until the last minute. In the past, nurses took everything from you that was removable, but now physicians and nurses want the patients to be as normal as possible—talking, hearing, seeing until just before the surgery. Glasses and hearing aids are labeled with the patient's name and returned right after the surgery.

If your contact lenses are disposable, throw them away in pre-op. Bring your glasses, because you may not feel well enough to put contacts in your eyes the first few days.

The anesthesiologist will talk to you about the history of any previous surgeries you may have had. If you had trouble with nausea or vomiting, this is the time to speak up, because the timing of your antinausea medicine can be changed. If you take the medicine prior to surgery rather than after you have your first bout with nausea, you won't get as sick or possibly you won't get sick at all. If this is your first surgery, but you easily get carsick or seasick, you might be a candidate for the antinausea medicine. Talk to the anesthesiologist about the possibility of this kind of prophylactic medicine; that is, medicine taken before it is needed to prevent something.

The anesthesiologist will place a needle in your arm to begin the intravenous fluids. You'll hear this referred to as an IV. The fluids are composed of a potassium and saltwater solution called saline. The purpose of the IV is to give you the fluids your body would normally have or need. If your doctor ordered it, the anesthesiologist will give you a dose of antibiotics prophylactically. Your IV will normally stay in until post-op Day 2 or 3, because it serves these additional important functions: to deliver extra fluids to bring down a fever, to deliver nutrition if you aren't eating well, and to deliver blood should you need a transfusion.

Just prior to surgery, I always come visit my patients. I follow several precautions: I tell my patients not to take anything for granted. I encourage them to write "THIS HIP" or "NO" on their skin with a felt-tip pen. As reinforcement, I hand-carry my patients' charts with me from my office to the operating room and I read them the morning of the surgery. I do everything possible before every surgery to ensure that no mistakes are made.

Someone from the surgical staff will pick you up from pre-op. They'll wheel you on your gurney into the operating room. If you're having general anesthesia, you won't remember much of this part, because the anesthesiologist will have already started giving you medicine to calm you and start to put you to sleep. (Occasionally people say they remember being moved from the stretcher to the operating table or they remember the overhead lights, but usually they don't.)

Some people get a regional rather than a general anesthetic. You and your doctor will determine which anesthesia will be best for you.

Preventing Blood Clots

There are inherent risks of undergoing surgery, and you need to discuss them with your doctor. There's a risk that you could have a negative reaction to the anesthesia. There's the risk of damage to the nerves or the blood vessels since we're working so close to them. There's the risk that your leg lengths could differ from each other after the surgery. There's the risk of infection. But of all the possible complications that can happen from surgery, the most important is a blood clot, because it can kill you.

When we talk about a dangerous type of blood clot, we're talking about a clot developing in a vein in either of your legs. It sits there and then all of a sudden—right after surgery, the next day, a week later, a month later, or three months later—it lets loose and throws itself into the bloodstream and flows up to the lung. The blood clot lodges there and blocks off a part of the breathing area of that lung. If it's a big clot, you can try to breathe all you want, but there won't be an exchange of oxygen and you could die.

A blood clot in a vein is called a **deep vein thrombosis (DVT),** while a clot that travels from one place to another is called an **embolism.** A clot that sticks in the lung is called a **pulmonary embolism.** No matter what they're called, we want to avoid all of them, so we take many precautions. We try to thin the blood immediately after surgery with an injected blood-thinner called heparin, or with a blood-thinner given by mouth called coumadin. There are pros and cons associated with each of these medicines, so talk to your doctor about which one he or she likes to use.

During surgery, we use various medications to keep a patient's blood pressure low, and we try to finish the surgery quickly. After surgery, we try to get the patient upright as soon as possible. We use pressurized stockings, which are placed on both your legs in the operating room and attached to an air pump machine. When the machine pushes air into the stockings, they gently squeeze first your ankles, then your calves, then your thighs. Then the air is completely released for a few seconds before starting the massaging effect again—ankles, then calves, then thighs. The stockings essentially refuse to let your blood stay stagnant. They push the blood out of the veins and keep the circulation going so the blood doesn't collect in the veins. Studies show that inflatable stockings prevent a large number of clots during the first seventy-two hours after surgery. Ask your doctor what his routine is or what his hospital staff does.

After hip surgery, you'll have swelling in your ankle, your knee, and maybe your whole leg, because we've blocked the normal flow of fluids upstream. The swelling could last for days, weeks, or even months. During that time, you'll probably want to buy some support stockings to help manage the swelling.

Pillows

By the time most people have hip surgery, they're usually already comfortable with a pillow between their legs as they sleep, so the introduction of such a pillow shouldn't be an intrusion. The staff in the operating room will strap your legs around the triangular-shaped abduction pillow to protect your hip while you're being moved (see Photo 65, page 150). The pillow keeps your legs apart in a stable position to prevent dislocation. This pillow is usually kept in place around the clock for two full days, then a regular pillow replaces it. Or you can choose to continue using your abduction pillow.

You may decide that you want the comfort of a pillow from home. If you do bring your own pillow, put a colored pillowcase on it, something that will distinguish it from the hospital's pillows. Without something to make it look different, your pillow could easily get mixed up with the hospital's.

Patient-Controlled Analgesia (PCA)

Patient-controlled analgesia is a device that's preprogrammed by your physician and attached bedside to the IV. It allows you to administer pain-killing drugs directly into your own IV. The program is set for a specific quantity of medicine that can be administered only once every preset time period, say every eight or ten minutes. Ask your surgeon if he recommends your using the PCA.

Day of Surgery: In Your Room

From the operating room, you'll be taken to the recovery room. The nurses there and your anesthesiologist will decide when it's time for you to be moved to your hospital room for the rest of your stay. Your IV will still be in place. You'll probably be given a few more doses of antibiotics through it.

The anesthesia can give you a dry mouth and a feeling of being dehydrated. Some patients aren't nauseous at all from the anesthesia and are hungry right after surgery. They can actually start eating in the recovery room. Most patients, however, will start with liquids first, then advance fairly quickly. Their first meal might be dinner the same evening of surgery.

Your bed will have a frame around it and a trapeze overhead. The trapeze is a bar you can grasp with your hands so you can use your arms to help adjust the position of your body. As you progress, you'll use it getting in and out of bed.

Every hospital is different. Some have private rooms, others have two or more patients per room. Some have cable TV, some don't. Do your research well ahead of surgery if those details concern you. You'll want to avoid a major surprise during the crucial days of recovery in the hospital.

Right after surgery, the nurses will ask you to do some ankle pumps: they'll say, "Push your toes away, then pull them back toward your head." They want to make sure you have control of your muscles and that all of the nerves are functioning. Also, ankle pumps help blood flow in the legs.

You'll need to take some deep breaths to keep your lungs working well. The number-one reason why some people have a fever right after surgery is a collapse of the small airways in the lungs. That collapse can cause a fever that could lead to pneumonia if not managed correctly. You need a good expansion of your lungs, and just being told to breathe deeply isn't enough. An **incentive spirometer** is a device created to motivate patients to breathe deeply. Essentially it's a plastic toy. You'll use your own breath to move three balls to the top of the device and hold them there a few seconds. You get visual feedback about how deeply you can breathe and hold that deep breath. You'll do that several times an hour whenever you're awake. It's a wonderful way to keep your lungs clear following the anesthesia required for surgery. If using a spirometer isn't a normal part of your hospital's routine, make sure they provide it for you.

Post-op Day 1

It's important to me that I see my patients early the next morning, and I'm hoping your surgeon will do the same. When I make **rounds** (visits to all my patients in the hospital), I spend time with the patients going over exercises they can do in bed. I explain how important it is for their brain to start talking to their muscles right away. Don't think of this time in bed as being "flat on your back," but as time you can use. You've been flexing and pointing your feet. Now you can start gently bending and straightening your knee ever so slightly. Keep trying to move the leg, and soon you'll no longer be afraid of moving it. If you watch TV, do these movements during the commercials, and the repetitions will add up. Then you won't be so wobbly when you stand up to walk, because your brain has already been communicating with your muscles.

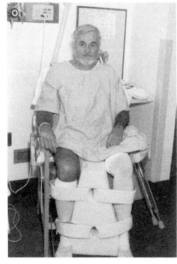

Photo 66. Post-op Day 2, sitting in a high chair with abduction pillow in place.

Before lunch, the therapists will help you up to try to sit for thirty to forty minutes, and will place the abduction pillow between your legs for safety even while sitting. (See Photo 66.) Recently, a master carpenter and I designed the Care Chair, which we use for postoperative hip patients at Cedars-Sinai Hospital. It makes life easier for postsurgical hip patients, because it reduces the amount of energy a patient needs to expend when sitting or standing. It provides a safe seating environment, because it encourages proper hip and knee positioning. A simple lever extends or retracts the footrest for ease and comfort.

Surgery is a premeditated trauma to the body. All the structures that have been cut—the skin, the muscles, the tendons, and the bone—need time to heal. We know which movements could interrupt the healing at the deep, medium, and surface levels, so specific hip precautions were developed to protect you from making those movements.

At the deepest level, your hip joint, once like a lightbulb screwed into a socket, is now more like an egg resting in a tablespoon. Until your body has had six weeks to go through the biological process of rebuilding the joint capsule with scar tissue, you don't want to move in such a way that would risk the dislocation of the ball from the socket.

As we close the tissues following surgery, the muscles, tendons, and fascia are overlapped and held together with sutures. However, those sutures are as weak as thread; they aren't worth anything in terms of structural strength. By following the hip precautions until these tissues have fused, you won't be pulling on the repair sites where the sutures hold the muscles together. Even the incision site on the surface of your

Hip Precautions
- Do not let your ankle or knee cross the midline of your body.
- Avoid hip flexion of more than 90 degrees.
- Don't combine hip flexion with internal rotation as shown in Photo 67.
- Don't stand with your feet turned inward.
- Don't rotate toward your postsurgical side as shown in Photo 68.
- Avoid lying or sitting on anything low, because you will put your hip at risk when trying to get up.
- Don't bend to pick up something from the floor.
- When in bed, don't reach way forward for a pillow or the covers.
- If your soap falls in the shower, don't bend to pick it up. Have several extra bars handy or buy a soap-on-a-rope for your six-week recovery.
- Use a high toilet seat so you won't hyperflex your hip when standing up.

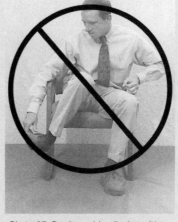 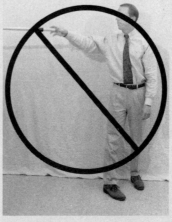

Photo 67. Don't combine flexion with internal rotation (assumes the right leg is the surgical leg).

Photo 68. Don't rotate toward your postsurgical hip (assumes the right leg is the surgical leg).

skin needs protection. If you make movements that tug on the skin, it may seep a clear fluid and delay the healing process. You want to keep the incision area dry for fastest healing.

All the precautions must be carefully followed for six weeks following surgery.

Although you may wish to do nothing but rest, your physical therapists will have specific goals for you even this first day after surgery. They will help you sit up on the edge of your bed and dangle your legs over the side. Next they'll help you stand and balance on crutches or a walker. Most people will start with a walker the first day and graduate to crutches when they feel less wobbly or nauseous. You'll be putting weight on your postsurgical hip the day after surgery.

If you managed sitting and standing relatively easily, you'll next be directed to take a few steps on your walker or crutches to the nearby chair. Practicing this maneuver from the bed to the chair is called transfer training. You'll sit in the chair for thirty to forty minutes, then transfer back into bed. If you don't make it into the chair on the first try, the therapists will do everything possible to see that you make it on the second try later in the day. The success of your surgery will be that much greater the sooner you get going.

Weight Management

One of my patients told me recently, "I wish I'd lost more weight before surgery. I intended to lose thirty pounds, but didn't get serious about it until I resigned my job the last month beforehand and then I got rid of ten pounds. Now, three days after surgery, I can feel that I'm putting twenty pounds too much on that new part in my hip. I'll get rid of the weight in the next few months and I'll be able to move around easier."

—*Robert Klapper, M.D.*

The Rest of Your Hospital Stay

Use pain medication if you need it. This isn't the time to turn it down. You'll probably need the medication in order to accomplish the physi-

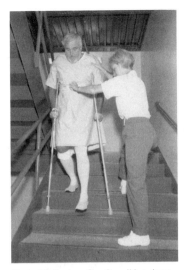

Photo 69. Post-op Day 2, walking down stairs with crutches.

cal tasks that are asked of you. You need to get out of bed, sit, and walk. Each day you'll do more, including going up and down stairs (Photo 69). If you say no to pain medication, then aren't able to do any of the physical therapy because it causes too much pain, you're defeating the whole program. Ask for painkillers as you need them. As the pain from surgery subsides and you're able to move with less pain, you won't need them as often.

The occupational therapist will begin teaching you how to accomplish the tasks of daily living without violating your hip precautions. She'll show you how to bathe or shower and how to use the long-handled devices that help you put on your shoes and socks. Any concerns you have about functioning in your home environment will be discussed, and she'll help solve those specific details.

You *could* go home as early as Day 4 or Day 5. In order to be discharged, however, you have to have achieved certain goals. If you live alone, you must be able to perform all of the functions by yourself. If you have someone at home who can help you, you have to be able to do them with minimal assistance.

You'll be evaluated to see whether you meet the criteria for discharge. Assuming you do, your dressing will be changed just before you leave the hospital. You'll leave the dressing on until you visit your surgeon in his office, usually a week later.

Going Home

Before you can go home, the therapists will make sure you can get out of bed by yourself and can walk to the bathroom and more than one hundred feet alone, and that you understand the precautions well. You'll also need to be able to walk up and down however many steps you'll be dealing with at home. If it's time for you to leave the hospital, but you're not doing these things, arrangements will have to be made for you to go to a rehabilitation facility such as a skilled nursing unit where patients don't need medical attention, but focus on doing intensive physical therapy twice a day while they have someone cooking their meals and caring for them in a nursing setting.

Once you arrive home, a physical therapist or an occupational therapist will visit to see if there are any ways to make your home more efficient with your temporary limitations. If they see anything of concern, they'll make adjustments. Their goal is to make your home a safe environment. They may suggest you put your written hip precautions in a prominent place—on your nightstand or dressing table as a reminder throughout the day.

I'm a big believer in taking vitamin C to promote healing. Increased doses of vitamin C (2000 mg. per day) accelerate your recovery. You or your surgeon may have other ideas regarding diet and nutritional supplements that will best help you heal and stay healthy.

One to two weeks later, you'll return to your doctor to have the staples along your incision removed. At that same time, seek approval to begin a pool program. You don't have to wait six weeks to start. I'm comfortable letting my patients go into the pool about two weeks after surgery. In the water, you'll be able to perform many safe movements that are still difficult on land. The sooner you start moving, the sooner you'll gain strength to make those same movements against gravity's force on land.

Driving after Surgery

How long before you can drive again depends on which hip had the surgery and on what kind of car you drive. If it was your left hip and the car you drive is not too low to the ground (a sports car) or too high (a sport utility vehicle) and has an automatic shift, you'll be driving a lot sooner than if you had the operation on your right hip and you drive a sports car. It takes longer to feel comfortable driving a stick shift.

Recovery Timeline

Every patient's recovery from surgery is unique. It's hard to give exact times for recovery, because much depends on how you answer these questions: How is your general medical health? What is the condition of your other hip? Your back? Your knees? Was there a leg-length problem? Each patient is different, but you will probably return to most, if not all, of your favorite activities. Here are some of the guidelines I suggest to my patients. Discuss your specific case with your surgeon.

- *Stitches removed.* This usually happens ten days to two weeks after surgery. As soon as the stitches or staples come out, you can get into the pool (see Chapter 7).
- *Two to six weeks.* For the first two weeks after you go home, you'll probably be using two crutches. You'll slowly progress to using only one crutch, then finally a cane. By the end of six weeks you should be able to walk without assistive devices.
- *Six to eight weeks.* You can generally play golf by now.
- *Three months.* You should be at the point where most of the pains from surgery are waning in your muscles and bursae. You may have a morning when you wake up and don't think of your hip as your first thought of the day.
- *Six months.* By now you're far away from the surgery in many ways. You're feeling good about being able to participate in your normal activities.
- *One-year anniversary.* In most cases, this is what your hip is going to be like from now on. There won't be many changes anymore. The scar tissue has evolved: it has healed, broken down, and healed again, finally making functional scar tissue that allows you to move well.
- *Lifetime.* Your new hip needs to be watched, even when it's working well for you. Your surgeon will most likely want you to come for regular checkups every six months or every year. Over 90 percent of the patients with hip implants are still doing well fifteen or twenty years later, and we expect some of the newer implants we're using to last up to thirty years. Just how long any implant will last depends on the bone, the implant, and the patient.

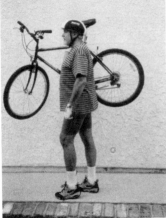

Photo 70. Two months after implant surgery.

You elected to undergo implant surgery for various reasons: to return to your athletic or sexual activities, to sleep without pain through the night, or to be able to walk well again, among other concerns. Disability in a hip joint causes possibly the most severe life limitations of all joint dysfunctions. When you're able to return to your normal life with a hip joint that functions fully without pain, your days will feel like a legitimate miracle. The implant will make a huge difference in the quality of your life. If you decide to choose this option, it's a large undertaking, but one with great rewards. Of all the surgical procedures studied by researchers, the highest satisfaction rate comes from hip implant patients.

Your life will be returned to you to enjoy.

Glossary

abduct   To move a body part away from the midline of the body.

abduction   Movement away from the midline of the body. Applied to the hip, it means moving the leg out to the side.

acetabulum   Located in the pelvis bone, it is the socket side of the hip's ball and socket joint.

acute   Injury of recent onset.

adduct   To move a body part toward the midline of the body.

adduction   Movement toward the midline of the body. Applied to the hip, it means moving the legs together or even crossing one over the other.

ADLs   Activities of daily living.

agonists   Half of a muscle pair, the muscles that contract to perform movement.

anesthesia   A drug agent that causes the loss of sensation or consciousness.

anesthesiologist   A medical doctor who is certified as a specialist in the administration of anesthesia.

antagonists   Half of a muscle pair, the muscles that relax so that the *agonists* can perform their movement.

antalgic gait   Walking with a limp because of pain.

arthro   Latin for "joint."

arthroscope   A pencil-thin surgical instrument that allows the surgeon to view inside the joint by way of a miniature video system and to operate on the interior of the joint.

arthroscopy   Any surgical procedure that uses the arthroscope.

articular cartilage   Also known as *hyaline cartilage*, it is the smooth thin layer that covers the ends of bones and protects the bones against impacting forces. The body's natural shock absorbers.

atrophy   The shrinking in size of muscle tissue.

autoimmune disease When the body reacts against one of its own parts as if it were foreign. Rheumatoid arthritis is an autoimmune disease.

avascular necrosis The loss of blood supply to the hip joint, which results in the death of the bone on the ball side of the joint.

bilateral Pertaining to both sides of the body.

Biodex A computerized rehabilitation machine that is capable of detecting subtle differences in muscular strength. See also *Cybex*, a similar machine.

biomechanics Efficient, good form. The position, posture, stance, or alignment that helps the body perform any activity most smoothly, with the least effort or strain.

bursae The fluid-containing sacs that provide cushioning around joints.

bursal sacs A more inclusive name for the bursae.

bursitis Inflammation of any of the bursae.

chondral Pertaining to the cartilage.

chronic Persisting over a long period of time.

circumduction A circular movement at a joint. Applied to the hip, this requires that the thigh move forward, then sideways, then backward in a circular pattern.

collateral circulation Secondary vessels supplying blood to an extremity (arm or leg) through indirect channels.

congenital Present at birth.

contraindications Things you should not do for a particular condition.

coxalgic gait Walking with a limp due to hip pain.

coxa magna A larger than normal femoral head.

crepitus A creaking or crackling sound or sensation when moving a joint, a muscle, or a tendon.

CT scan Computerized axial tomography. A three-dimensional X ray that is 100 times more sensitive than an ordinary X ray.

Cybex A computerized rehabilitation machine that is capable of detecting subtle differences in muscular strengths. See also *Biodex*, a similar machine.

deep vein thrombosis (DVT) A blood clot within a vein.

embolism A blood clot that travels from one location to another within the body.

extension Straightening of a joint, or as applied to the hip, reaching backward with the leg behind the body.

fascia Bands of fibrous tissues throughout the body that surround muscles.

femur   The thigh bone, the largest bone in the body. The top of the femur is the ball part of the ball and socket that makes up the hip joint.

femoral head   The ball on the end of the femur or thigh bone.

fibrocartilage   The rubbery cartilage that composes the ears and the nose.

flexion   Bending a joint. As applied to the hip, lifting or pulling the thigh closer to the torso, or bending at the hip.

fracture   A break or crack in a bone or cartilage.

fronds   Points of inflammation inside a joint that hang down from the ceiling like stalactites.

functionability   A person's ability to function within his or her personal environment.

golgi tendon organ   A sensor imbedded deep in the tendon that responds to slow stretch by lengthening the muscle.

Heberden's nodes   Bony enlargements of the finger joints in osteoarthritis.

hyaline cartilage   Synonymous with *articular cartilage*. The shock-absorbing surfaces on the ends of bones.

incentive spirometer   A device given to a postsurgical patient that motivates him or her to breathe deeply. Visual feedback shows the depth and strength of each breath.

internist   A medical doctor certified in internal medicine.

isokinetic exercise   Exercise that is variable and based upon the patient's strength. As the patient pushes harder, the resistance increases proportionately.

isometric exercise   Exercise that does not involve any movement of the joint or limb, a fixed muscular contraction.

isometrically   Pertaining to the use of a muscle group that contracts but doesn't cause movement.

IV   Intravenous fluids given to supply nutrients the body needs.

joint capsule   The tough fibers and ligaments that encase the hip joint.

labrum   The fibrous rim that surrounds the hip joint.

lavage   Flushing out corrosive joint fluid with clear saline solution.

ligaments   Strong, fibrous tissues that link bones at a joint.

loose bodies   Fragments, usually of cartilage or bone, inside the joint.

meniscus   The shock-absorbing cartilage in the knee.

modality   A therapeutic agent applied to a patient to reduce pain and swelling while it arouses the body's natural healing mechanisms.

MRI   Magnetic resonance imaging. A diagnostic technology that uses a superconducting magnet and a computer to precisely display soft tissue and bone that is not apparent on X ray.

muscle spindle   Sensors in the belly of muscles that warn muscles to contract when they are stretched so they will retain their normal length.

musculoskeletal   The muscular and skeletal systems viewed as a whole.

NSAIDs   Nonsteroidal anti-inflammatory drugs.

orthopedist   A medical doctor who is a certified specialist in treating disorders of the bones, muscles, joints, ligaments, tendons, and other parts of the musculoskeletal system.

osteoporosis   A loss of calcium and bone density, usually associated with aging.

palpate   To examine by the sense of touch.

passive, sustained stretch   A manual technique applied by a therapist to increase range of movement.

pathognomonic   Specific to one thing only.

periarticular erosions   Defects and crevices around the perimeter of the joint where the cartilage stops and the regular bone begins, usually seen in rheumatoid arthritis.

phonophoresis   The use of ultrasound plus the addition of medicine to the water-based gel. The ultrasound thus drives the medicine through the skin into the underlying tissues.

placebo   A medicine given to appease the patient, but containing no true medicinal properties.

prehab   Rehabilitation done prior to surgery.

pre-op   Pre-operative, as in pre-op procedures and pre-op holding room.

prophylactic   Protecting or defending from disease, a preventive measure or drug.

pulmonary embolism   A blood clot that lodges in the lungs.

quadriceps   The four muscles that run down the front of the thigh causing hip flexion and knee extension.

radiologist   A medical doctor who is a certified specialist in the interpretation of X rays, MRIs, and CT scans.

reciprocate stairs   To place one foot on a stair, then the opposite foot on the next stair above, and continue alternating in this manner.

rehab   The conversational word for rehabilitation.

rehabilitation   Reconditioning of the musculoskeletal system to restore maximum function.

repeated contractions   A manual physical therapy technique that begins the strengthening process for weak muscles.

rheumatologist   A medical doctor who is a certified specialist in rheumatological diseases including rheumatoid arthritis, lupus, osteoarthritis, and fibromyalgia.

rounds   The common phrase for a doctor's visits to his or her patients in the hospital following surgery.

sacroiliac   The junction where the pelvis meets the spine.

saline solution   Salt water.

sciatica   Pain radiating down the sciatic nerve into the back of the thigh, the calf, and into the toes.

sclerosis   An uneven hardening of the bone due to unequal weight bearing in a joint.

spur   An abnormal bone growth at the edge of joints.

starting pain   A sure sign of hip joint problem; after resting, if pain is present upon starting to move, that indicates the problem stems from the hip.

stenosis   Narrowing of a canal or opening, often applied to a narrowing of the various openings in the vertebrae that pinch the nerves.

subchondral   Beneath the cartilage.

subcutaneous   Beneath the skin.

synovectomy   The removal of all or a portion of the inflamed lining of a joint.

synovial fluid   The lubricating fluid within the hip joint.

synovial lining   Synonymous with synovium, the lining of the hip joint.

synovium   The lining of the hip joint.

tendinitis   Inflammation of a tendon.

tendons   The fibrous cords of connective tissue that attach muscles to bones.

Thera-Bands   Latex bands used for resistance exercises.

vasoconstriction   Narrowing of the blood vessels resulting in a reduction of blood flow.

vasodilation   Enlargement of the blood vessels resulting in increased blood flow.

X ray   Electromagnetic radiation that passes through the body to create a picture of the dense tissues of the body, such as bone.

Appendix

The following is a list of manufacturers and their products that appeared in the text.

AquaJogger Low Impact Fitness

Excel Sports Science
P.O. Box 1453
Eugene, OR 97440
(800) 922-9544
(541) 484-2454
Fax: (541) 484-0501
email: info@aquajogger.com
Web site: www.aquajogger.com
Product: AquaJogger, DeltaBells, AquaJogger swimsuits

A flotation belt for deep-water exercise with special design for lower back support. DeltaBells are hand-held water exercise barbells. Swimsuit collection of durable bathing suits, unitards, and water wear.

Aquatic Trends Inc.

649 U.S. Highway 1
Suite 14
North Palm Beach, FL 33408
(561) 844-3003
Fax: (561) 844-0302
email: aquatictrends@flinet.com
Web site: www.aquatictrends.com
Product: Aquatrend Pool Exercise Bar

A removable device designed to attach to a home pool's skimmer box, offering hand holds for stretching and exercise.

Bioenergetics

200 Industrial Dr.
Birmingham, AL 35211
(800) 938-8378
(205) 941-2110
Fax: (205) 942-9723
email: Wetvest@Quicklink.net
Web site: www.wetvest.com
Products: Wet Vest, Wet Vest II, Wet Belt
   The first manufacturer of flotation vests and belts for deep-water exercise.

Huey's Athletic Network

3014 Arizona Ave.
Santa Monica, CA 90404
(310) 829-5622
Fax: (310) 828-5401
email: lyndahuey@aol.com
Web site: www.lahuey.com
Products: Waterpower Workout Tether, a Wet Belt made exclusively for
Huey's Athletic Network, *The Complete Waterpower Workout Book,* and "Lynda
Huey's Waterpower Workout" video.
   Tether holds you in the correct position for deep-water interval training.
H.A.N. model Wet Belt adjusts at both the front and back of the body.

HYDRO-FIT Inc.

1328 W. 2nd Avenue
Eugene, OR 97402-4127
(800) 346-7295
Fax: (541) 484-1443
email: hfproducts@aol.com
Web site: www.hydrofit.com
Product: HYDRO-FIT Buoyancy & Resistance Cuffs, HYDRO-FIT Hand
Buoys, Hydro-Fit Swim/Therapy Bar
   Cuffs can be placed on the ankles, wrists, upper arms, or around the waist
to supply buoyancy for deep-water exercise, or resistance for shallow-water
work. Hand Buoys and Swim/Therapy bar are used as support items during
deep-water exercise.

Hydro-Tone Fitness Systems, Inc.

16691 Gothard St., Suite M
Huntington Beach, CA 92647
(800) 622-8663
(714) 848-8284
Fax: (714) 848-9035
email: hydrotone@aol.com
Web site: www.hydrotone.com
Products: Hydro-Tone Belt and Hydro-Tone Boots

Ultra-buoyant black flotation belt for deep-water exercise, and high-resistance boots to put on feet for lower body exercises.

HydroWorx International, Inc.

29 Northeast Dr.
Hershey, PA 17033
(800) 753-9633
(717) 533-0916
Fax: (717) 553-0917
email: hydroworx@aol.com
Web site: www.hydroworx.com
Product: HydroWorx pools

Small pool for indoor institutional use. Pool bottom is a treadmill and is moveable from flush with the floor to six feet deep. Features jets, underwater video cameras, and computer programming.

KKC Inc.

12051 Forestgate Drive
Dallas, TX 75243
(972) 235-1033
Fax: (972) 235-9664
email: masinali@aol.com
Product: Hydra-Flow Water Weights

Soft cuffs around the shins for buoyancy and resistance.

NZ Manufacturing, Inc.

3502 C St., N.E.
Auburn, WA 98002-1702
Product: Waterpower Workout Tether
 Designed by Lynda Huey for in-place water running and walking.

Order from Huey's Athletic Network:

(310) 829-5622
Fax: (310) 828-5401
e-mail: lyndahuey@aol.com
Web site: www.lahuey.com

O'Neill Corp.

1071 - 41st Avenue
Santa Cruz, CA 95063
Inside California (800) 662-7873
Outside California (800) 538-0764
Fax: (800) 538-2085
email: oneill@oneill.com
Web site: www.teamoneill.com
Products: Wet suits, Thermo shirts, Thin Skins
 Clothing for warmth in cool water.

RoJo Rehabilitation

P.O. Box 3085
Del Mar, CA 92014
(619) 794-4867
Product: Care Chair
 A chair designed for safety and comfort for postsurgical patients.

Speedo Authentic Fitness

6040 Bandini Blvd.
Los Angeles, CA 90040
(213) 726-1262
Fax: (213) 720-4662
Web site: www.speedo.com
Products: Speedo Aquatic Exercise Belt and swimsuits
 Teal-colored flotation belt for deep-water exercise and several lines of
bathing suits.

SwimEx Systems

P.O. Box 328
Warren, RI 02885
(800) 877-7946
(401) 245-7946
Fax: (401) 245-3160
email: swimex@TPIcomp.com
Web site: www.swimex.com
Product: SwimEx pools

Small pool for indoor institutional or private use. Features multidepth platforms.

Tru-Fit

330 Lynnway
Lynn, MA 01901
(800) 592-6544
FAX: (781) 593-7602
email: info@tru-fit.com
Web site: www.tru-fit.com
Product: ICE/HEAT gel packs and cloth wraps with Velcro fastening so you can apply ice or heat to an injured area while having complete mobility.

Index

Note: **Bold type** indicates names of exercises.

About the Authors

Robert C. Klapper, M.D., likes to tell his patients: "My father was a carpenter and my mother was a nurse, so I was destined to become an orthopedic surgeon. The most important thing my father taught me was 'Measure twice, cut once.' It comes in handy every day I'm in the operating room."

This fits comfortably with Dr. Klapper's education and medical training (an art history degree from Columbia College, a medical degree from Columbia University's College of Physicians and Surgeons, an internship at Cedars-Sinai Medical Center, and a residency at the Hospital for Special Surgery in New York, followed by a fellowship in arthritis and implant surgery at the Kerlan-Jobe Clinic in Los Angeles) and with his bold, visionary research that has led to nine patents on instruments used to do complicated hip surgery. He is currently Director of Cedars-Sinai Orthopedic Associates at Cedars-Sinai Medical Center in Los Angeles. He has written articles for *Clinical Orthopedics and Related Research*, the *American Journal of Sports Medicine*, and other publications and was recently named orthopedic technical advisor to the television series *ER*. Of this role Dr. Klapper writes, "We have to work harder at letting people know what we do as surgeons."

Lynda Huey, M.S., starred as a sprinter at San Jose State University, earned both a bachelor's and a master's degree, coached track and field and volleyball at several universities, and wrote her autobiography, *A Running Start*, before she was thirty. Her second book, *The Waterpower Workout*, resulted from her pioneering work in developing water exercises for fitness and rehabilitation of athletic injuries; and her third book, *The Complete Waterpower Workout Book* (with Robert Forster, P.T.), details advanced programs for fitness enthusiasts, dancers, Olympic gold medalists, and postsurgical patients.

Huey hosted a radio sports show for National Public Radio throughout the 1980s and worked for NBC at the 1988 Olympic Games. She designed therapy pools and aquatic therapy protocols for hospitals and appeared on TV and radio as a world authority on water training.

Since 1983 Huey's Athletic Network in Santa Monica, California, and, more recently, her Total Aquatic Rehab in Los Angeles have cross-trained and rehabilitated elite athletes and entertainers, including Paula Abdul, Gail Devers, Florence Griffith Joyner, Jackie Joyner-Kersee, Mike Powell, Cybill Shepherd, Sinbad, Barbra Streisand, Wilt Chamberlain, and others.